Epidemiology of Natural Disasters

Contributions to Epidemiology and Biostatistics

Vol. 5

Series Editor
M.A. Klingberg, Ness-Ziona/Tel-Aviv

Coeditor
C. Papier, Tel-Aviv

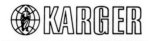

S. Karger · Basel · München · Paris · London · New York · Tokyo · Sydney

Epidemiology of
Natural Disasters

J. Seaman
Save the Children Fund, London

With contributions by
S. Leivesley
International Disaster Institute, London

C. Hogg
Appropriate Health Resources Technology Action Group, London

19 figures and 11 tables, 1984

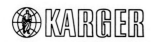 KARGER

S. Karger · Basel · München · Paris · London · New York · Tokyo · Sydney

Contributions to Epidemiology and Biostatistics

John Seaman

Senior Overseas Medical Officer, Save the Children Fund (U.K.), 17 Grove Lane, London S.E.5 8RD (England)

Sally Leivesley

International Disaster Institute, 85 Marylebone High St., London W1M 3DE (England)

Christine Hogg

Appropriate Health Resources Technology Action Group, 85 Marylebone High St., London W1M 3DE (England)

National Library of Medicine, Cataloging in Publication
Seaman, J.
Epidemiology of natural disasters/J. Seaman, S. Leivesley, C. Hogg. – Basel; New York : Karger, 1984
(Contributions to epidemiology and biostatistics; v. 5)
Includes index.
1. Disasters 2. Disaster Planning 3. Disease Outbreaks – prevention & control II. Leivesley, S. (Sally) III. Hogg, C. (Christine) IV. Title V. Series
W1 CO778RC v. 5 [WA 105 S438e]
ISBN 3-8055-3779-4

Drug Dosage

The authors and the publisher have exerted every effort to ensure that drug selection and dosage set forth in this text are in accord with current recommendations and practice at the time of publication. However, in view of ongoing research, changes in government regulations, and the constant flow of information relating to drug therapy and drug reactions, the reader is urged to check the package insert for each drug for any change in indications and dosage and for added warnings and precautions. This is particularly important when the recommended agent is a new and/or infrequently employed drug.

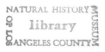

Contents

Acknowledgements

The authors are indebted to many people for their assistance in the preparation of this book. Particular thanks are due to Professor *Marcus Klingberg* and Ms. *Cheri Papier* for much helpful criticism and for their assistance in preparing the text for publication; to Dr. *Frances D'Souza* and Dr. *Robin Stephenson* of the International Disaster Institute for providing much of the literature on which the text is based; to *John Rivers* of the London School of Hygiene and Tropical Medicine for help with the chapter on environmental exposure, and to Mr. *Tony Jackson* of Oxfam for providing literature on food relief after the 1976 Guatemala earthquake. Thanks are also due to Mrs. *Joan Elliot* for patiently typing the several drafts of the text.

The authors also wish to thank Blackwell Scientific Publications, Dr. *Roger Glass,* Dr. *L.E. Mount,* Dr. *Alfred Sommer,* Dr. *Karl Western* and the editors of the *Bulletin of the Pan American Health Organization, Disasters, The Lancet* and *Science N.Y.* for granting permission to reproduce various figures in the book.

Foreword

Disasters, seen as large-scale disruptions of human ecology, represent a major health problem in the deaths, casualties and suffering which they cause. Doubtless, in the future their importance will increase even further in the wake of population explosion, technological development and social or political upheavals. The last decade has seen significant changes in the health management of disasters, whether natural or man-made. It is increasingly appreciated that the phenomenon goes far beyond the punctual provision of relief to the population affected and extends from advanced preparedness to the problems of long-term rehabilitation. Media reports and better communications have stimulated public pressure for more effective disaster aid. Both governmental and the non-governmental international agencies which have always been pivotal in disaster relief have seen the need for a more integrated approach to the subject, using the large body of knowledge which has been accumulating through case studies and exercises in the evaluation of disasters. Disaster epidemiology is a newly emerging discipline which attempts to develop a systematic approach to the measurement of the health effects of disasters, aiming at a more efficient matching of needs and resources.

This highly topical book will be useful to all those concerned with the health problem represented by disasters, from the field worker or the member of a rescue team after an earthquake, to the official in charge of predisaster planning and the management of relief. It successfully draws together the many aspects of disasters which can contribute to management. At a time when more and more health professionals are showing an interest in disaster work, this book elucidates the differences between the population approach and the individual approach and so helps to solve the conflicts they generate.

Conveying so much information in so few pages, with the right mix of scientific data and human concern, in a practical and clear format, is no mean achievement. It is the result of the many years of field work and study of disasters by *John Seaman,* most recently as editor of the journal *Disasters.* It also reflects the experience of the London Technical Group, founded in 1971, now the International Disaster Institute.

I am convinced that this book will directly contribute to reducing the suffering of those many millions of our fellow human beings who will be exposed to disasters in the years to come.

Prof. *Michel F. Lechat,* Bruxelles

Introduction

The effects of disasters are often obvious. No complex analysis is required to know that disasters may kill and injure many thousands of people, or that they may leave large populations homeless or without food. But while the vulnerability of populations of the richer countries has declined, that of the developing world has increased through population growth, urbanisation and pressure on land; despite the apparent simplicity of the relationship between disasters and the health of populations, problems still regularly arise with the effective provision of relief.

Worldwide, disasters are very common events and enormous sums are spent on disaster relief and reconstruction. It is estimated that disasters involving international assistance occur on average once a week [15]; although it is impossible to calculate the exact sums spent on relief, as no central records are kept, one estimate suggests that emergency relief, from international and local sources combined, now consumes approximately $ 1 billion each year [10].

The 'epidemiology of disasters' finds its origins in the massive international relief operation mounted during the civil war in Nigeria in the late 1960s. The war caused food shortages which affected, to a greater or lesser extent, a population of several million people in a wide area. As relief supplies were limited, it was necessary to discriminate between those who were genuinely in need of food and those who were not. Through the involvement of epidemiologists from the US Center for Disease Control and from the Quaker Relief Service, techniques were developed for the rapid assessment of nutritional status, and surveys were conducted to identify the population in need [1, 5, 9].

Since then, progress in the 'epidemiology of disasters' has been uneven. Most studies have been made on the causes and effects of food shortage on populations in the developing world. Techniques developed during the crises in the West African Sahel, Ethiopia, Bangladesh and Uganda [3, 6, 8, 12, 14] have become a routine part of relief work in famine areas and in refugee populations.

Much less information is available concerning the effects of the more violent types of disaster, such as earthquake, cyclone, tornado and flood, on the health of populations. In a literature review in 1972, *Western* [15] could find only two papers published prior to the Nigerian civil war where the epidemiological method had been consciously applied to these types of disasters. Since then, perhaps only a dozen more studies meeting this description have been added to the literature.[1]

Western [15] advanced three main reasons for the lack of information on disasters. First, the study of disasters has tended to follow narrow specialty lines. Although many aspects of disasters have been intensively studied, and some, such as the geophysics of earthquakes, have led to considerable advance in understanding the causes of natural catastrophe, there is no academic specialization with an interest in their effects on populations. Most studies of the medical aspects of disasters have been conducted by physicians and other medical workers who become involved by engaging in relief work.

Second, many aspects of disasters and perhaps particularly those covered by this book are, by their nature, difficult to study. The lack of time in which to organise an investigation, the reluctance of relief workers to keep records, the movement of populations from and within disaster areas, and many other factors, work against accurate and complete observation.

Lastly, most relief agencies concerned with disaster – and there are estimates that these now number several hundred worldwide – regard relief as an entirely operational affair. Many administrators refuse to acknowledge that useful generalisations may be drawn from experience of the effects of disasters and the types of relief which may be useful in future relief operations. Medicines, clothes, shelter, food and medical personnel may be despatched to any disaster area with an assurance that they will be

---

[1] Most of these studies have been conducted by epidemiologists from the US Center for Disease Control, Atlanta, Ga. Only two other centers have had a sustained interest in the subject: the Center for Research on the Epidemiology of Disasters, School of Public Health, University of Louvain, Bruxelles, Belgium, and the International Disaster Institute, London, UK.

required. As a result, few agencies have been prepared to accord a high priority to systematic observation and record-keeping, and much valuable experience has been lost.

Definitions of Disaster

There have been many attempts to define the world 'disaster'[2], none of which is entirely satisfactory. They are either too broad, so that trivial events might be included, or too narrow, so that exceptions could easily be found. We suggest that no effective formal definition is possible, or even required. The term 'disaster' is often used to cover such disparate events as wars, industrial accidents, blizzards, avalanches, volcanoes, earthquakes, fires, famines and many types of windstorms and floods – events which have little in common except for their destructiveness.

Disasters are often classified into two groups, 'natural' and 'man-made', and are sometimes subdivided again into those of 'slow' and 'sudden' onset. These headings are descriptively convenient, but do not form a satisfactory classification of either the immediate causes or the effects of different agents or communities. Some types of disasters – such as fires, may be 'natural' or 'man-made' according to circumstances. Some 'sudden-onset' disasters such as floods, may occur rather slowly under some conditions, and the 'slow-onset' disaster of famine – or at least the abrupt termination of food supplies to part of a population – may be very sudden indeed, as the market price of food rises out of reach of the poor [13]. 'Natural' disasters may be the direct result of human actions, for example, through the siting of settlements in areas of known risk to flood, or the use of construction methods known to be of high risk in earthquakes. As sociologists have often pointed out, natural events such as earthquakes

---

[2] For example: '. . . . the relatively sudden and widespread disturbance of a social system and life of a community or a large part of a community by some agent or event over which those involved have little or no control' [2];

'. . . . an event (or series of events) which seriously disrupts normal activities' [4];

'More sociologically, a disaster is an event, located in time and space which produces the conditions whereby the continuity of the structure and processes of social units become problematic' [7];

'A disaster is an overwhelming ecological disruption occurring on a scale sufficient to require outside assistance' [11].

and floods are not intrinsically dangerous; it is the relationship between the natural agent and people that makes them so.

In this book, a more restricted classification of natural disasters has been used, including only earthquakes, cyclones and storm surges, tornadoes, tsunamis, floods and volcanoes. The reasons for this are two-fold: first, these types of disasters are responsible for most disaster-related loss of life, particularly in developing countries, and second, because they are the main concern of the international relief organisations. While other types of events such as blizzards and forest fires may be no less 'disasters' to an affected community, they are mainly of interest to local relief agencies, including usually the fire service and the police, and they do not fall easily into the same descriptive framework. Drought and famine have been excluded on the grounds that they raise wholly different issues in terms of cause, effect and relief; therefore, they should not be included in the same classification of 'disasters' at all [see also chap. 4, p. 89].

Sources of Information on Disaster

In a very complete review of the sources of information relevant to the epidemiology of disasters, *Western* [15] divided them into those dating before 1945 and those after 1945. As he pointed out, several factors make it difficult to compare the earlier with the more recent literature.

(a) *Changes in living conditions.* The population explosion, urbanisation and differing economic conditions in various regions of the world have created differential risks to populations. In some rich countries, the vulnerability of populations to certain types of disaster has been substantially reduced by measures such as flood control works and the enforcement of building standards in areas of high earthquake risk. In much of the poor world, the reverse has occurred; the exponential rise in the population of some cities, the pressure on land and the steadily deteriorating economic conditions of both governments and individuals have forced increasing populations into more hazardous zones.

(b) *Medical progress during the past 30 years.* Improvements in hygiene, vaccines, antibiotics and other drugs, have practically eliminated the scourges which were associated with disasters in the past (e.g. typhus, relapsing fever and plague). Such epidemics are now restricted to isolated epicentres and pose little threat after most calamities.

(c) *Improved communications and transport.* With the introduction of the jet engine and cheap electronic devices, it is now possible for the outside world to hear of and respond to a disaster in remote parts of the world within a few days at most.

(d) *Increased interest.* Before World War II, the international relief agencies were few in number. Most international relief was channelled through Red Cross agencies. Since then, the economic boom in the western countries has led to both a greater knowledge of conditions in the developing world and to much greater opportunities for action. The period has seen the creation of the United Nations technical agencies, including one (UNDRO) with a specific responsibility for disaster-related activities, the growth of bilateral aid and the creation of a considerable number of private charitable groups, many of which have an interest in overseas disaster relief.

Contemporary sources of information on natural disasters span a wide range, from press reports, reports from governments, United Nations and independent agencies, to articles in the technical and scientific press. The total contemporary literature relevant to disasters, not including the technical literature on geophysics and meteorology, must now run to some hundreds of thousands of documents. We have been very select in our use of this literature, partly because many agency and government sources are simply not available for inspection, but mainly because of the poor quality and biases of the literature itself. Few documents, for example, give more than a summary description of the nature of the specific disaster with estimated numbers of dead and injured, before passing on to a list of relief requirements and material delivered; even fewer give any details of the sources of the information presented. Most agency material is written in such a way as to put the work of that agency in the best possible light. Even in the technical press, much of the literature is concerned with descriptions of technique (e.g. hospital planning, rescue), usually without any reference to any actual experience of disaster.

The Aim and Scope of the Book

For the reasons mentioned, very little of the information contained in this book was obtained by formal epidemiological enquiry. This book is an attempt to apply the epidemiological method, using that term in its broadest sense, to existing information, rather than a review of epidemiological research in its more usually-accepted form.

The topics of the six main chapters of this book are: death and injury, communicable disease, environmental exposure, food and nutrition, psychological response, and application of epidemiological methods to disasters. In the final chapter, the implications for disaster planning and conducting relief operations are discussed. These topics are dealt with at very different depths, reflecting the extent of the published literature on each topic. The discussion has been limited to the period immediately after disaster, as almost nothing has been published on the longerterm effects of disasters on health.

References

1 Arnhold, R.: The QUAC stick: a field measure used by the Quaker Service team, Nigeria. J. trop. Pediat. 15: 243–247 (1969).
2 Beach, H.D.: Management of human behaviour in disaster (Department of National Health and Welfare, Canada 1967); cited in Western [15].
3 Beillik, R.J.; Henderson, P.: Mortality, nutritional status and diet during the famine in Karamoja, Uganda 1980. Lancet ii: 1330–1333 (1981).
4 Cisin, I.H.; Clark, W.B.: The methodological challenge of disaster research; in Baker, Chapman, Man and society in disaster (Basic Books, New York 1962).
5 Davis, L.E.: Epidemiology of famine in the Nigerian crisis: rapid evaluation of malnutrition by height and arm circumference in large populations. Am. J. clin. Nutr. 24: 358–364 (1971).
6 Dodge, C.P.: Practical application of nutritional assessment – malnutrition in the flood area of Bangladesh, 1974. Disasters 4: 311–314 (1980).
7 Dynes, O.R.; Quarantelli, E.L.: Helping behaviour in large-scale disasters – a social organizational approach. Disaster Research Center, rep. 91 (Ohio State University, Columbus 1975).
8 Hogan, R.C.; Broske, S.P.; Davis, J.P.; Eckerson, D.; Epler, G.; Guyer, B.J.; Kloth, T.J.; Kloff, C.A.; Ross, R.; Rosenberg, R.L.; Staehling, N.W.; Lane, J.M.: Sahel nutrition surveys, 1974/1975. Disasters 1: 117–124 (1977).
9 Lowenstein, M.S.; Phillips, J.F.: Evaluation of arm circumference measurement for determining nutritional status of children and its use in an acute epidemic of malnutrition, Owerri, Nigeria, following the Nigerian civil war. Am. J. clin. Nutr. 26: 226–233 (1973).
10 National Research Council: The US Government disaster assistance program. Report of Commitee on International Disaster Assistance (National Acadamy of Sciences, Washington 1978).
11 Pan American Health Organization: The health management of natural disasters (Pan American Health Organization, Washington 1980).
12 Seaman, J.; Holt, J.; Rivers, J.: The effect of drought on human nutrition in an Ethiopian province. Int. J. Epidemiol. 7: 31–40 (1978).
13 Seaman, J.; Holt, J.: Markets and famines in the third world. Disasters 4: 283–297 (1980).

14 Sommer, A.; Mosely, W.H.: East Bengal cyclone of 1970 – epidemiological approach to disaster assessment. Lancet *i:* 1029–1036 (1972).

15 Western, K.A.: The epidemiology of natural and man-made disasters – the present state of the art; thesis University of London (1972).

1. Death and Injury

Introduction

In the popular press, the prominence given to any disaster depends mainly upon the numbers of people killed or injured; much less upon the extent to which an economy or society has been disrupted. With few exceptions, disaster relief agencies have also tended to reflect the same scale of values. Large reported death tolls tend to elicit massive support from abroad in terms of medicine, equipment and medical personnel. For example, within 2 weeks of the 1976 Guatemalan earthquake, over 120 tons of drugs had arrived from abroad; the task of sorting and classifying these had not been completed several months after the impact [42, 69]. This is perhaps the most well-documented case, but similar examples can be found in the lore of almost any major disaster.

Most commentators on the medical aspects of disaster relief have also tended to assume that major disasters lead to large needs for medical assistance. There is now a large literature on the medical aspects of disaster relief. The greater part of this literature is taken up with descriptions of the organisational aspects of relief such as hospital planning, the management of mass casualties, suitable types of medical supplies and the most effective administrative procedures to be adopted [47]. Few commentators have asked the fundamental questions: 'What are the effects of disasters on human populations?'; 'Who is killed?'; 'Who is injured?'; and 'How does this vary among disasters of different types in different areas?'. In other words, 'What is the problem with which medical relief is actually concerned?'.

In this chapter, an attempt has been made to summarise the present knowledge regarding the relationship between common types of natural disaster and human death and injury, and to see if this knowledge can contribute towards a more rational approach to disaster prevention and relief.

Sources and Quality of Data

We have relied mainly upon the published literature, supplemented, when available, by government and international agency reports. Data relevant to health effects of disaster are not only scarce, but are often of suspect quality.

Several sources of difficulty arise. For example, official government and agency statistics make up the major bulk of available data on crude numbers of deaths and injuries. These statistics are of variable quality. In some instances, particularly for relatively easily enumerated aspects such as deaths, they may be reasonably accurate. They may be based upon complete body counts, and in large areas, sometimes obtained through area-by-area counts. Major flooding may result in the dispersal of corpses, making official statistics no better than guesses. In some cases, the government may not issue any statistics at all. For example, the much-quoted figure of 650,000 deaths (according to some commentators, one million) in the 1976 Tang-Shan earthquake, has not, so far as we can tell, been confirmed or denied by the Chinese government. Official statistics on 'injury' may be even more suspect, as the term is rarely defined and may encompass many diagnoses, including routine medical and obstetric cases. Sometimes data may be sound (e.g. statistics on admissions to a single hospital) but may represent only part of a larger data set.

In general, data from the developing countries are of poorer quality than those from the industrialised world. Population censuses in developing countries may not be accurate to within hundreds of thousands; in any case, they may change seasonally through migration. Therefore, it is only rarely possible to express findings in terms of statistical rates.

This review has been limited to cover earthquakes, destructive winds, storm surges, tsunamis and floods. We have excluded disasters such as war, and events such as train crashes and industrial accidents which are often classified as disasters. These events do not fall into the same classification as 'natural' disasters, either in terms of their effects, or in terms of the issues they raise about prevention and relief. Volcanoes have been excluded from the main description because of the relative rarity of this type of 'disaster' and because of the wide range of effects seen from one volcano to another in various parts of the world. This topic has been summarized in the Appendix.

Earthquakes

Earthquakes occur in well-defined belts and are thought to result from interactions at the edges of great plates which make up the surface of the world. Nearly all earthquakes directly affecting human populations occur in a narrow ring around the Pacific basin, in the eastern USSR and much of China, along the 'sundra arc' through New Guinea, and across the Mediterranean and Trans-Himalayan zones. Australia, southern India, West, Central and South Africa, and most of Asia are relatively free of seismic activity. However, no area is immune to the risk of earthquakes. Some earthquakes causing great loss of life, such as the 1960 Agadir earthquake in Morocco, and the 1967 Koyna earthquake in India, have occurred well away from zones of high seismic activity.

Thousands of minor earthquakes occur each year, although only a small proportion of these result in loss of life. No reasonably complete listing of mortality from earthquakes appears to have been compiled, except in a few countries such as the United States, Japan and Iran. Figure 1 shows the frequency distribution of mortality in one series of earthquakes occurring during the period 1903–1978 in Iran. It should be noted that this is a period which has been marked by changes in both population density and, to some extent, building style.

Nevertheless, it is clear that the impact of earthquakes in terms of mortality varies enormously from place to place. During this century, the continental United States has suffered only three earthquakes which have resulted in deaths of over 100 people [2], whereas some countries, including China, Turkey, Iran, Italy and several Central and South American countries have suffered repeatedly from earthquakes with death tolls in the thousands. Some poor countries, such as Ethiopia and Papua New Guinea, although often affected by earthquakes, have suffered only slightly in terms of resultant death and injury.

Variations in mortality rates among different countries are primarily due to differences in building styles and density of settlements. The over-

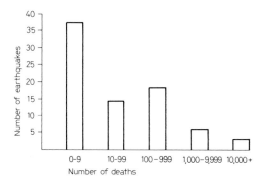

Fig. 1. Frequency distribution of deaths from 78 earthquakes in Iran during the period 1903–1978. Data obtained from Berberian [9].

whelming majority of people who die in earthquakes are killed by the collapse of man-made structures, particularly domestic dwellings. However, building damage is only one of several variables found to influence the pattern of death and injury following earthquakes. For descriptive purposes it is convenient to divide the subject under four main headings: (1) the seismic and geologic features of an area, the building design and construction, and specific aspects of building construction and the risks to occupants; (2) the location of inhabitants (e.g. indoors or outdoors); (3) the age and sex of inhabitants and those killed or injured; (4) the types of injury, severity and timing of presentation for treatment.

Seismic and Geologic Features of an Area and Building Design and Construction; Specific Aspects of Building Construction and the Risks to Occupants

The relationship between earthquake and structural failure is complex and is beyond the scope of this book. However, as it is of importance in considering the causes of earthquake mortality, a summary of the major variables is given here.

Seismic and Geologic Features of an Area and Building Design and Construction

Damage to buildings from earthquakes generally occurs because of horizontal forces exerted against buildings which are designed to resist vertical forces, or because of the uneven resistance of structural elements to destructive forces. According to *Iacopy* [32], four seismic and geologic factors strongly influence damage to man-made structures: (1) the strength of the earthquake waves reaching the surface, particularly the horizontal component; (2) the duration of the earthquake motion, as the cumulative effect of a series of tremors is the usual cause of wall collapse; (3) the proximity of a structure to a fault or fault zone; (4) the geologic foundation, considered by many engineers to be the most important factor in earthquake damage.

The importance of each of these factors to building damage varies widely from place-to-place and time-to-time and among earthquakes of different intensities and durations. *Nichols* [52] describes a number of cases where damage to buildings was confined to, or much worse in, buildings which were located on alluvial deposits rather than firmer ground. The Caracas earthquake of 1965, for example, measuring 6.5 on the Richter scale, caused heavy damage only to structures built on alluvial deposits. Four high-rise buildings collapsed in pancake fashion, killing 200 people, and a number of other buildings were rendered uninhabitable. The selective nature of the damage appeared to be due to the coincidence of the fundamental period of ground movements within the alluvial deposits, and the fundamental wave period of high-rise buildings between 10 and 20 stories, creating a harmonic oscillation of the buildings affected [62]. Similar cases have been noted in Turkey, Japan and the Philippines [52].

However, in those earthquakes occurring during the past decade which have caused more than 2,000 deaths[1], considerations of the subtleties of geology, siting and engineering are of less interest: these earthquakes have all occurred in areas characterised by a building style which is both prone to structural failure even in modest tremors and is of particular danger to occupants during collapse. Although varying considerably, the buildings in these areas are generally made of mud, mud-brick or rock with little wood or concrete reinforcement.

In many areas of Central and South America prone to seismic activity, most dwellings are built of adobe (mud-brick) roofed with tile or corrugated iron. In Iran, mud is also widely used as a building material. *Saidi* [58], writing of the effects of the 1962 earthquake, which caused some

---

[1] Turkey – Lice, Van and Gediz; Guatemala; Nicaragua – Managua; Peru; China – Tang-Shan; Iran – Qir and Tabas-E-Golshan; Algeria – El Asnam; Italy – Campania/Basilicata.

12,000 deaths in the area west of Teheran, described the housing in the affected area: 'Dwellings are simple and uniform; houses of one, and rarely two storeys shelter families and livestock. The walls of houses are thick layers of dried mud, roofed over by crossbeams of medium-sized tree trunks covered by a thinner layer of mud and large twigs.'

In eastern Turkey, traditional dwellings are built of adobe brick, cobblestone or unshaped basalt blocks. Very few cobblestone or field-stone houses survived the Varto earthquake of 1966, and most casualties resulted from the collapse of roofs or walls of heavy materials [72]. Similar observations apply to the Lice earthquake of 1975 in eastern Turkey [41]. The Gediz (Turkey) earthquake of 1970, which killed more than 10,000 people, destroyed or badly damaged approximately 9,528 dwellings and caused lesser damage to another 17,000 [51]. In this region, Mitchell identified four basic types of construction [51]: cobble (field-stone) or adobe wall bearing; braced frames of hand-hewn timber (or round posts); tile or brick walls; and reinforced concrete, although many houses were of hybrid design. This hybrid construction reportedly accounted for the largest number of deaths from the Gediz earthquake, 'when walls disintegrated and tons of rock and mud collapsed into living areas'.

Reports of other earthquakes in the Mediterranean area also suggest that older, traditional buildings were at greatest risk during the earthquakes in: Sicily, 1968 [29]; Skopje, Yugoslavia, 1963 [10]; Friuli, Italy, 1976 [31]; and the recent earthquake in southern Italy, near Naples, in 1980 [63].

As already noted, the impact of an earthquake in terms of building damage is not simply a function of distance from an earthquake's epicentre. Housing damage, such as in the Caracas earthquake described previously, may be selective due to specific characteristics of design, location and geological foundation. But in areas where the major determinant of damage is the design and method of construction of the buildings themselves, the patterns of building destruction and of death and injury may be closely related to the location of the epicentre or to the movement of a fault line.

The Tabas-E-Golshan earthquake in Iran (1978), which killed more than 20,000 people, affected an area in which the vast majority of buildings were of adobe or rock and mud mortar. A study by *Berberian* [9] showed that the pattern of destruction presented a clear correlation with the fault line. Damage and destruction of highest intensity (80–100% destruction and 50–85% casualties) were experienced for approximately 80 km along

Table I. A comparison of the effects of the earthquakes in Managua, Nicaragua (1972) and in San Fernando, California (1971): data from *Kates* et al. [36]

Earthquake characteristics and effects	Managua, 1972	San Fernando, 1971
Magnitude (Richter scale)	5.6	6.6
Duration of strong shaking, s	5–10	10
Area of Mercalli intensity[a]		
VIII–XI, km^2	66.5	500
VII–VIII, km^2	100	1,500
Estimated		
Population of affected area	420,000	7,000,000
Dead	4,000–6,000	60
Injured	20,000	2,540
Houses destroyed or unsafe	50,000	915[b]

[a]The Mercalli scale of earthquake intensity ranks earthquakes from 0 to XII according to the subjective experience of individuals and physical damage to structures.
[b]This figure includes 65 apartments.

the ground rupture and roughly 3 km on either side of it. Severe damage stopped about 45 km from the ground rupture.

A similar pattern of destruction and death related to a fault line was observed in the 1976 Guatemalan earthquake [23]. The massive destruction in central Managua in 1972, caused by a relatively small earthquake, was related to the site of the city (see table I). It is transected by at least five faults, of which four ruptured during the earthquake. No part of the city is more than 0.5 km from a fault line. The earthquake destroyed most adobe and non-reinforced concrete building sites over the faults, and ground-shaking destroyed many more in adjacent areas [11].

In some areas, landslip may represent an additional hazard. Hundreds of mainly slum houses built on ravines around Guatemala City were thrown to the bottom, together with their occupants, during the 1976 earthquake [57]. The 1970 earthquake in Peru [13]: 'triggered off a series of massive rock falls, screes and landslides. Houses and fields located beneath unstable cliffs were either buried or severely bombarded by rocks, and a large number of vehicles in the busy Sunday afternoon traffic were battered to destruction with their passengers.'

Figure 2 shows the relationship between the number of houses destroyed and mortality in a series of Turkish earthquakes between 1912

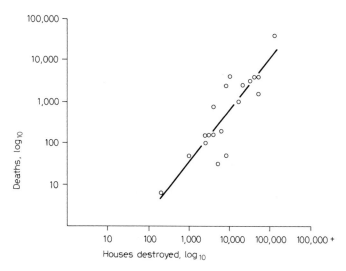

Fig. 2. The relationship between mortality and number of houses reported destroyed in 19 Turkish earthquakes during the period 1912–1976. Sources: *Altay* [1]; *Ilhan* [33]; London Technical Group [41].

and 1976. The correlation (r) between the number of houses destroyed and mortality in this series is 0.88. In the Tabas-E-Golshan earthquake in Iran (1978), the correlation between the percentage of building damage and the percentage of the population killed in 74 villages, calculated from data given by *Berberian* [9] was 0.76.

A comparison of the 1976 earthquake in Managua and the San Fernando Valley earthquake of 1971 (table I) illustrates the relative vulnerability of populations employing different standards of construction to earthquakes of similar magnitude. Other features of these earthquakes differ, such as population density and the time of day at which the shock occurred, and the comparison is only approximate. A more powerful earthquake striking this area of California might well produce mortality comparable to that seen in Guatemala. Projections, based on shocks 100 times the strength of that of the 1971 earthquake, suggest that mortality might be expected to be in the range of 10,000 to 1,000,000 depending on the time of day and other conditions [5].

While most earthquakes causing substantial mortality have occurred in developing countries, it should be noted that this is not directly a function of poverty. Several seismically-active developing countries experience little damage or mortality as a result of earthquakes. For example, the traditional Ethiopian village hut as well as many urban buildings are constructed of mud and wattle, often on a substantial timber frame, and are earthquake resistant [26]; Papua New Guinea employs similar safe structures for the most part. In Bali, traditional building techniques directed specifically at earthquake resistance have been described [38].

Specific Aspects of Building Construction and the Risks to Occupants
To the best of our knowledge, only one study has been conducted regarding the relationship between specific aspects of building design and construction and the risks to the occupants from the earthquake. This study was conducted by *Glass* et al. [23] following the 1976 earthquake in Guatemala, which killed 23,000 and injured approximately 76,000 people. The study was conducted in the village of Santa Maria Cauque, located approximately 30 miles west of Guatemala City. At the time of the earthquake, the village had a population of 1,577, housed mainly in one-room shelters made either of adobe block or cornstalk, roofed with thatch, tile or corrugated iron. The earthquake, which registered 7.5 on the Richter scale, occurred at 3.05 a.m., when the villagers were asleep, and lasted 39 s. It was not preceded by warning shocks and people were unable to take refuge even within buildings. All the buildings of the village were destroyed, with the exception of the school, the town hall, the health clinic, and one house – all of which were made of reinforced concrete. Casualties included 78 people killed and 38 seriously injured (for definition, see p. 20). Systematic enquiry by *Glass* of 259 out of the 277 heads-of-households showed that all of the deaths and serious injuries occurred in adobe houses. While all but one of the non-adobe houses collapsed, none of them caused major injury or death. No relationship was found between death or injury and room or house size, the number of doors and windows, number of members of family, or the location of people within a room at the time of the earthquake. Those close to the corners, unsupported walls, or under door jambs, appeared to be at as great a risk as others. Of the housing characteristics examined, only the age of the adobe blocks showed a significant relationship with trauma; adobe houses more than 7 years old showed a 1.6-fold increase in risk to the occupants. Surprisingly, all injuries or deaths were attributed to falling adobe, and none to roofing materials. The socioeconomic status of a family was found to be correlated with house size but not with severity of injury.

Location of Inhabitants (Indoors or Outdoors)

As most earthquake trauma is caused by the collapse of buildings, the location of people with respect to buildings at the time of impact would be expected to show a relationship with the number killed or injured. In cases of preceding foreshocks, which are heeded by the population, lives may be saved. The earthquake in Managua on December 23, 1972, was preceded by shocks at 10 p.m. on December 22. As a result, some people slept outside and were spared the three major shocks during the early hours of the following morning [36]. Many similar examples could be cited.

Lomnitz [40] catalogued a long series of earthquakes in Chile, and found a close relationship between mortality and time of day at which the earthquake occurred. He attributed the diurnal variation in earthquake mortality to a combination of human factors, but mostly to the periodicity of dwelling occupancy. He cited *Goll* [25] as saying of the Chilean population: 'The inhabitants avoid bodily harm by escaping from their homes because of any moderately perceptible shaking, since there is no telling what might follow . . .'. This pattern of behaviour is still observed today, according to *Lomnitz*.

One pattern of mortality might be expected for those who work in fields or in other open air occupations; another pattern for those who work in offices or factories. The San Fernando earthquake of 1971 occurred in the early morning before the commuter rush. The collapse of a freeway overpass killed 2 persons. The number might have been much higher had the earthquake occurred 2 h later during the rush-hour [53].

Narrow streets may pose other risks for those leaving a building. It was reported that in the coastal towns of Peru in 1970 [13]: 'People who had rushed instinctively out into the wide streets at the first tremors escaped unscathed; many of those trapped in the collapsed houses with flimsy roofs were able to be rescued. In contrast, the people in the (mountainous) Callejon de Huaylas who reacted similarly to the first tremors were immediately buried in the narrow streets by tons of rubble bursting out from both sides under the weight of heavy town roofs.' In the parish of Venzone, hit by the 1976 Friuli earthquake, *Hogg* [31] noted that 'agile groups suffered more than the elderly or very young.' This is because they ran out into the streets which unlike those of modern towns are especially narrow, and were crushed by falling masonry' (see also age- and sex-specific mortality).

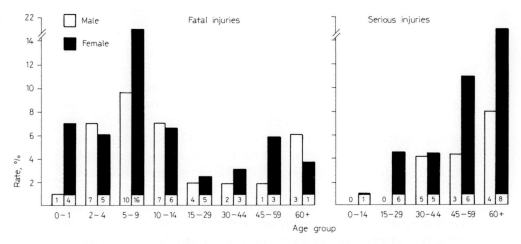

Fig. 3. Age- and sex-specific rates for serious injuries and fatal injuries in Santa Maria Cauque. Numbers in bars represent absolute numbers of injuries. Reproduced from *Glass* et al. [23].

Age and Sex of Inhabitants and Those Killed or Injured

Little reliable data are available on the impact of earthquakes on different groups within a population, although the available evidence suggests that it may strike different groups in a very selective way. The published data, of which we are aware, are restricted to studies conducted after the 1976 Guatemalan earthquake in three villages; some more general data from Managua, from Venzone (a parish of Friuli in Italy); and from the Ashkabad (1948) and Tashkent (1966) earthquakes in the USSR.

The survey by *Glass* et al. [23] in the village of Santa Maria Cauque, gave age- and sex-specific rates for death and serious injury in that population. 'Serious injuries' were defined as 'those patients who required hospitalisation or an outpatient follow-up of more than two weeks, and included major fractures (n = 30), severe contusions (n = 4) and open wounds (n = 4)'. Mortality rates were found to be high for the very young and the very old, but relatively low for those aged 15–44 years (see fig. 3). It was also found that infants under 1 year of age had lower mortality rates than their older siblings. The risk of death to the youngest child (the last born) was lower than that to the next older sibling. The risk of death was greatest in the penultimate child and decreased thereafter with increasing

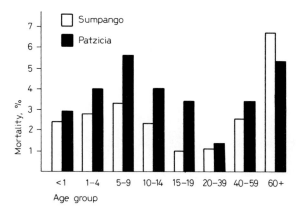

Fig. 4. Age-specific mortality in two towns in Guatemala. Sumpango – 244 deaths in population of 10,232; Patzicia – 377 deaths in population of 10,850. Data from published histograms in *de Ville de Goyet* et al. [70].

age, with the risk to the oldest child (the first born) being the least. *Glass* attributed this penomenon to the fact that the youngest child normally slept with its mother and was therefore protected. It was found that the youngest child generally shared the fate of the mother, with both surviving (n = 28) or dying (n = 5), versus the mother dying alone (n = 1), or the child dying alone (n = 1).

A similar pattern of age-specific mortality was noted in two Guatemalan villages affected by the same earthquake [71] (fig. 4), after the Managua, Nicaragua earthquake of 1972 [23], and in the two examples for the USSR. Of those who died in the 1948 Ashkabad earthquake, 47% were women and 18% were men. In Tashkent (1966) there were 25% more women casualties than men [7].

A different pattern of age-specific mortality was noted by *Hogg* [31] in Venzone (see fig. 5). There, a relatively higher mortality is evident in an older age group (45–54 years). This she attributed to the escape from houses of the more agile members of the population, who were then killed by falling masonry in the streets.

The frequency of major injury recorded by *Glass* et al. [23] in Guatemala increased steadily with age (fig. 3). Only 7 out of a total of 38 seriously injured were under 29 years of age, and the risk of injury was consistently greater in women than men in almost all age groups. This pattern *Glass* noted, is similar to the age/sex distribution of hip fractures

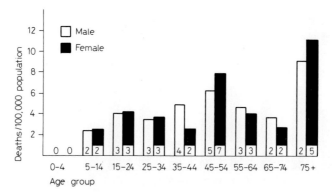

Fig. 5. Age-specific mortality in Venzone, Friuli, Italy in the 1976 earthquake. Numbers in bars represent absolute numbers of deaths. Data from *Hogg* [31] calculated using population data from Friuli-Venezia-Giulia for 1976 given in reference 55.

in the United States, which occurs preferentially in elderly and post-meno-pausal women because of their weakened osteoporotic bones. No informa-tion is available on the age- and sex-specific rates of injury or death from other earthquakes.

Types of Injury, Severity and Timing of Presentation for Treatment

Types of Injury

Patients seen at hospitals and other treatment centres provide the only published statistics available on types of injury sustained in earthquakes. These data are admittedly biased even for the severely injured. The term 'injured', although freely used in earthquake reports, has never been properly defined. It may include, as in Guatemala [70], almost any kind of medical complaint regardless of cause. However, practically nothing has been recorded specifically about the types and relative frequencies of minor injuries seen after earthquakes.

In tables IIa and IIb, data are presented from the seven published examples in which casualties attending medical facilities are analysed by type. All of them present data under different diagnostic headings and each represents a different post-earthquake period. The findings from the Lar (southern Iran) earthquake of 1960 are for 85 seriously injured patients transferred to a hospital in Shiraz [58]. The patients from Jalapa

Table IIa. Types and percent of injuries (fractures) recorded following the earthquakes in Managua, Nicaragua (1972), Bali (1974), Guatemala (1976) and Iran (1962)

Managua		Bali[1]		Guatemala		Iran[2]	
Hand	6	upper extremity	3.9	upper extremity	3.2	upper and lower extremities	57.6
Wrist	4	lower extremity	18.8	lower extremity	6.4	vertebrae	11.8
Forearm	8	spine	3.9	clavicle	11.5	pelvis	8.2
Elbow	2	other causes	73.4	pelvis	2.5	injury to face and head	10.6
Humerus	7			other causes	76.4	chest injury	11.8
Hip	4						
Femur	7						
Knee	5						
Tibia	9						
Ankle	9						
Foot	10						
Clavicle	10						
Spine	6						
Pelvis	8						
Face and jaw	6						
Nb. of patients approximately	300		202		157		85

Data from Leimina [39], Saidi [58], de Ville de Goyet and Jeanée [71] and Whittaker et al. [76].
[1] Patients were admitted to hospital by day 3 after the earthquake.
[2] A further 26 cases were classified as 'minor injury, dehydration and gastroenteritis'.

(Guatemala) were referred for X-ray to the Jalapa hospital [70]. The data collected by Whittaker et al. [76] in Managua and the Ashkabad (USSR) findings [7] are probably the most useful. The former are representative of patients presenting for primary triage, and the latter of those with all categories of earthquake injuries. In San Fernando (1971) the reasons for hospital attendance are given in detail: but this earthquake, in an area of highly developed services and very different building styles may not be easily compared with the other examples. The data from the Bali earthquake of 1974 which caused 573 deaths, refers only to those patients admitted to hospital [39].

The data presented in table II suggest that fractures make up a large part of the casualty load and that the site of fractures is fairly evenly distrib-

Table IIb. Types and percent of injuries recorded following the earthquakes in San Fernando, Calif. (1971), Ashkabad, USSR (1948) and Tashkent, USSR (1966)

San Fernando				Ashkabad	Tashkent
	hospital admissions	out-patients			
Lacerations	–	57.8	soft tissue injury	31.8	–
Contusions	–	10.5	long bone fracture	17.3	21.1
Abrasions	–	7.8	head injury	15.0	36.7
Fractures	53.3	23.9	spinal injury	5.0	3.4
Head injury	24.8	–	pelvic injury	4.0	0.0
Burns	14.3	–	thoracic injury	4.0	–
Back injury	7.6	–	injury to abdominal		
			organs	0.2	–
			other injuries	22.7	38.8
Number of patients	105[1]	1768[2]	Approximately 4,000		Unknown

Data from *Beinin* [7] and *Olsen* [53].
– = The category of injury is not mentioned.
[1] The classification of 110 further admissions was: cardiac = 41; psychiatric = 26; general medical = 8; remainder = 35.
[2] The classification of 560 further out-patients was: emotional reaction = 210; cardiac = 140; remainder = 210.

uted around the body. The suggestion by *de Ville de Goyet* et al. [70] after the Guatemalan earthquake that fractures of the clavicle may be particularly common after earthquake is only partly supported by the findings in Managua where clavicle fractures represented 10% of all fractures. After the Ashkabad earthquake it is reported, in additon to the data presented in the table, that fractures of the clavicle and scapula combined accounted for 9% of all fractures seen [7]. Severe injuries not involving fractures, or additional to them also appear to be common.

Long [43] reports that internal injuries were predominately ruptured bladders and injuries to the urinary tract. This he attributes to the occurrence of the earthquake at 3 a.m. when people's bladders were full.

Whittaker et al. [76] noted after the Managua earthquake that most of the casualties were crush-type injuries: 'The patients showed severe swelling of an involved extremity, blister formation and various degrees of nerve involvement manifested by absent sensation and motor function.

Usually the circulation was intact . . . in contrast to more ordinary types of trauma, the fractured bones were almost of secondary importance . . .'. Despite this, he could not fully document the renal failure aspect of the 'crush syndrome'[2] as patients were not retained at the hospital for a long enough time. One patient with severe crush injuries of the legs, who was in shock on admission, was observed to pass dark-brown urine, an indication of myoglobinuria. *de Ville de Goyet and Jeannée* [71]found no documented cases of crush syndrome after the Guatemalan earthquake in spite of repeated enquiries. In contrast, the syndrome appears to have been sufficiently common after the 1960 Agadir earthquake that a clinical series of 22 cases of varying severity could be conducted from a group of 429 of the injured evacuated to Casablanca [50]. In Ashkabad, crush syndrome was noted in 3.5% of all earthquake injuries [7]. We have found no other record of crush syndrome from the recent literature on earthquakes. It is not clear whether this lack of information reflects the real absence of the syndrome or merely a lack of observation. There appear to be no features of the Agadir or Ashkabad earthquakes markedly different from other earthquakes in similar areas, so we suspect the latter to be the case.

Severity of Injury

Of those injured in earthquakes, the overwhelming majority sustain minor injuries, or injuries requiring only out-patient treatment. In Ashkabad, the ratio of 'severe' to 'light' injuries is reported as 1:9.4, and in Tashkent, 1:15.9 [7]. In Khorasan, Iran (1968) the ratio of in-patients to out-patients treated was 1:29.6 [48], and in San Fernando, 1:17 [53]. Although the information in most papers reviewed is incomplete, it is implied by the scale of the total casualty load that only a minority of patients required admission to hospital.

Timing of Presentation at Treatment Centres

This factor is clearly of importance when considering the provision of emergency assistance. Admissions to the US field hospital (fig. 6b) which was deployed at Chimaltenango, Guatemala on the 4th day after the 1976 earthquake rose rapidly on the first day of operation, reached a peak on the second operational day and fell off rapidly thereafter; a second smaller

---

[2] Compression of a limb for several hours, as can result from being trapped under rubble, causes muscle damage and results in (a) oedema of the damaged area, haemo-concentration, lowered blood pressure and shock, and (b) the release of products of muscle damage, such as myoglobin which appears in the urine and may cause renal failure [12].

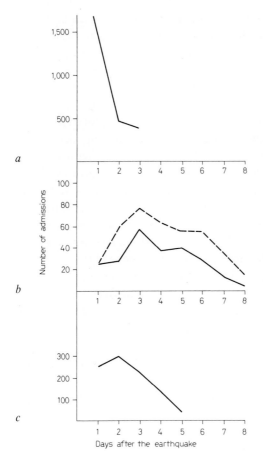

Fig. 6. Numbers of patients admitted to hospitals on successive days following three earthquakes. *a* San Fernando 1971 – all admissions and hospital out-patients. Data from *Olsen* [53]. *b* Chimaltenango, Guatemala 1976 – number of admissions (solid line) and bed occupancy (broken line) in percent, to US field hospital. Data read from published graph in *de Ville de Goyet* et al. [70]. *c* Managua, Nicaragua 1972 – patients admitted to US emergency tent hospital. Data from *Whittaker* et al. [76].

wave of admissions was due in part to the increasing efficiency of the relief operation in bringing casualties from outlying areas. Communications had been severely disrupted during the first few days after the earthquake and the total number of hospital beds available was reduced due to the closure of several hospitals following a severe after-shock [70]. Admissions to the emergency tent hospital in Managua in 1972 (fig. 6c) show a similar sharp rise and fall, but over a shorter period [76]. In San Fernando (fig. 6a), an area well served with transport and hospitals, the pattern of admissions shows a still sharper rise and fall [53].

A question asked by *Glass* et al. [23] in Santa Maria Cauque concerned the effect that a better and faster rescue service might have had on mortality. He found that 6 people (7%) of those who died remained communicative until dawn, 3 h after the earthquake, but were not rescued because of the darkness of the night and the distance between houses.

Cyclones[3] and Tornadoes

Cyclones and tornadoes do not form a homogeneous group of events when considering deaths and injuries. Like earthquakes, they occur in relatively circumscribed areas of the world, areas with very different geography and patterns of human settlement. In the case of cyclones, the damage caused by winds is often compounded by floods from heavy rain and by the violent innundations known as storm surges. In this section we have concentrated on those examples in which damage, death and injury resulted directly either from (1) cyclones uncomplicated by flood or storm surge, or (2) those in which the effects can be reasonably clearly separated. This division is somewhat arbitrary; reference should also be made to the section on floods (see p. 39). We have found no useful account of death or injury resulting from other types of destructive winds.

Cyclones

Cyclones begin as low pressure areas – the 'depression' of temperate zone weather forecasts – in equatorial latitudes. As warm moist air is drawn tangentially into the area of low pressure, the system is sustained and intensified by the release of heat from condensation at higher altitudes. The form of a tropical cyclone has been made familiar from satellite photographs as a great spiral of cloud some 500 km across, with a central calm 'eye'. The most severe winds occur in a circular band surrounding the eye, where gusts of 240 km/h may occur. Wind speeds diminish from the centre to the periphery, although surface winds of up to 64 km/h may occur 160 km from the centre.

---

[3] Called 'hurricanes' in the Caribbean and Western Atlantic and 'typhoons' in the Western Pacific; in meteorological terms they are identical.

As cyclones are formed over the sea and rapidly dissipate as they pass on to a continental land mass, their effects are felt mainly by seamen, and by populations in coastal areas. Cyclones show a seasonal variation in occurrence in different parts of the world.

Relatively little has been published on death and injury from cyclones. Indeed, it is doubtful if mortality from some of the less damaging cyclone strikes in India and Bangladesh has been recorded at all. Average loss of life in the USA during the period 1955–1969 from hurricanes (cyclones) is given at 75 per year [74]. Descriptions of two reliable accounts follow.

The 1974 Darwin Cyclone Disaster. At midnight on December 14, 1974, Darwin, the capital of Northern Territory, Australia, with a population of 45,000 was struck by the tropical cyclone Tracy. Enormous damage was done to the town; 90% of all houses were destroyed or seriously damaged, and only 500 houses remained continuously habitable [49, 75]. Wind speeds were reported up to 150 mph. (240 km/h). 49 people were killed, the majority from 'crush asphyxia' [75]; 140 were seriously injured and approximately 1,000 received minor injuries. Casualties began to present at Darwin Hospital when the wind dropped soon after dawn, and most of the 500 patients seen had presented by early afternoon [27]. Some hundreds of patients received treatment at peripheral first-aid centres. 112 patients were admitted to hospitals on the first day [75].

Of those patients treated as out-patients, the great majority suffered from lacerations caused by flying glass and other debris, with a few 'closed fractures and other injuries'. No burns were seen [27]. Of those admitted to hospital, roughly half had severe lacerations and half had injuries from missiles, crushing or falls, while some had both types of injury [27]. A breakdown of diagnoses in admitted patients is given by *Gurd* et al. [27].[4] 35 theatre cases were treated at Darwin hospital.

A policy of primary suture of wounds was adopted; some patients were seen subsequently with wound infections. One man developed tetanus after a forehead laceration was sutured with a piece of wood *in situ*. 'Quite a number' of accidental injuries, mainly penetrating wounds of the feet,

---

[4] Penetrating wound of abdomen, 1; penetrating wound of chest, 1; bilateral amputation of feet, 1; other severe lacerations, 60; paraplegia, 5; other spinal injuries, 7; fractured pelvis, 6; major head injuries, 2; closed abdominal injuries, 3; other blunt trauma, 50. Multiple diagnoses were made on some patients.

were incurred after the cyclone during the clearing and searching of the rubble [27].

Hurricane Liza, Baja, Calif. At 4.00 p.m. on October 1, 1976, hurricane Liza struck Baja, Calif. Maximum wind velocity recorded was 165 km/h with 20 cm of rain falling in 7 h. The population of the area was approximately 130,000 of whom 60,000 lived in the town of La Paz. When a 4-metre high dam gave way, 450 people were killed; virtually all of them died in the flood. 405 bodies were recovered, but no reliable estimates could be made of individuals missing because of the unregistered population of low-income immigrant workers.

'Serious injuries were conspicuous by their absence' [73]. In La Paz, there were no injuries sufficiently severe to require hospitalisation. Two hundred out-patients were treated; minor injuries consisted of cuts, abrasions and bruises. The only major trauma resulted from a bus crash after the hurricane.

Other Cyclones. Other accounts of the effects of tropical cyclones give at best only a simple enumeration of the number of dead and injured, without further detail, e.g. hurricane Beulah, September 21, 1967, in which 18 people died in southern Texas, and over 8,000 were injured [54]. There is even less information about 'smaller' cyclone disasters in poorer countries. The cyclone which swept the Island of Masirah, Oman, in June 1977, killed 2 persons and injured 48. The torrential rains which fell on the adjacent Dhofar Province killed a further 103, although it is not clear if the flood, wind or the collapse of houses was responsible [64]. The November 1978 cyclone in Sri Lanka, which in terms of loss of life and damage to property was probably the most serious in the island's history, is reported to have killed 915 people [66]. This cyclone was accompanied by a storm surge of modest proportions, but it is again unclear how many deaths resulted from the cyclone, the collapse of houses or drowning. An UNDRO report [66] states that within the 35-km belt of high winds, roofs were blown off about 50% of buildings. The buildings in one area which had brick or concrete walls, were mostly left intact. In some instances, however, collapsing roofs pulled down walls with them. In rural areas, houses of light construction were completely destroyed. A large proportion of houses with mud walls were also destroyed when the wind removed roofs and heavy rain washed away the walls. Some buildings in all areas were destroyed by falling trees. Scattered deaths from drowning were reported in some areas subject to heavy rainfall. In the Sri Lanka cyclone handbook [61], Resstler stated that 'there were not a large number of severely injured patients in relation to the extent of property damage', and that 'the injuries most commonly seen were lacerations, fractures and bruises; severe injuries were compound fractures, spinal injuries, head injuries and severe crush injuries . . .'.

The causes of death and injury during the 1979 David and Frederick hurricanes in Dominica and the Dominican Republic are also unclear [67, 68]. Total mortality was approximately 2,000 with a further 4,000 injured. In at least one instance, over 100 people were killed when the church in which they were sheltering, collapsed [68].

Tornadoes

A tornado is like a cyclone, a vortex of air, but on a much smaller scale. Although the mechanism of formation of tornadoes is still poorly understood, it is thought that they begin with small, weak vortices formed as air flows around buildings and other obstacles. Once established, the vortex is strengthened and maintained by a flow of warm air up the centre of the spiralling column. Small tornadoes are well known from all continents as 'dust devils' but it is only in some countries and at some seasons that they reach a seriously destructive size.

Most published accounts of tornadoes and tornado damage are from the United States, although the USSR, Japan, Bangladesh, China, Australia, Bermuda and Fiji have also published reports [65]. In Bangladesh, for example, a report describes a tornado in Noakhali, a provincial town, which killed 70 people and injured 5,000 [37]. Even in Britain, over 400 tornadoes have been recorded during the past two decades. In June 1967, tornadoes killed 20 people in France, Belgium and the Netherlands [35]. In the USA, tornadoes show a strong seasonal variation in frequency, most occurring between April and July during the late afternoon.

The velocity of the air rising in the centre of a tornado vortex may be very high and is responsible for much of the damage caused as objects – cars, even railway stock – are 'vacuumed' from the ground[5]. The sharp pressure difference across a tornado may cause houses to 'explode' as the outside pressure abruptly falls. A tornado can cause destruction

[5] However more recent research has challenged this view [35]; tornado damage may result mainly from aerodynamic lift caused by high speed wind movements across roofs, rather than from the pressure difference.

500–1,000 m wide as it moves along its track. When crossing an urban area, it may cut a swathe of almost total destruction through houses and other buildings.

Descriptions of Five Tornadoes. Several good and detailed accounts of the effects of tornadoes are available from the American literature: the Worcester tornado (June 9, 1953); Topeka (June 8, 1966); the Indiana tornadoes (April 11, 1965); Dallas (April 2, 1957); and Wichita Falls (April 10, 1979). As these events are very similar, only a summary account of each will be given.

(1) Worcester Country: 4.30 p.m. June 9, 1953 [4]. In central Massachusetts, a tornado tracked south for 1 h over a course 35 miles long and from 200 yards to half a mile wide across rural areas and suburban and densely populated parts of the city of Worcester. Almost every building in the path of the tornado was demolished, including factories, but mainly single dwellings of middle-class people. In the city of Worcester alone, more than 8,000 people were in the track of the tornado. During its entire course, the tornado covered ground on which more than 20,000 people lived. 94 people were killed, 85 of them outright; 490 suffered injuries requiring hospitalisation and in addition there were more than 1,000 minor injuries. No effective warning was given in any area, and few people had knowledge of impending disaster. Some had even gone outside in order to look at a heavy shower of hailstones.

(2) Dallas: 4.30 p.m. April, 2, 1957 [20]. This tornado originated in southwest Dallas and moved northwards at 25 mph, cutting a continuous path 100 yards wide for approximately 16 miles. Many structures in the path of the tornado were demolished explosively. 10 people were killed, and 183 required hospital treatment. As the tornado was visible throughout its course, many people were forewarned of its approach.

(3) Indiana: 8.10 p.m. April 11, 1965 [46]. Three tornadoes struck the state of Indiana causing approximately 140 deaths. One tornado struck near the town of Lebanon (approximately 30 miles northwest of Indianapolis) killing 17 people immediately. 24 patients were admitted to two local hospitals and a further 37 were treated as out-patients.

(4) Topeka: 7.15 p.m. June 8, 1966 [6]. This tornado travelled at 35 mph and carved a path 22 miles long and a quarter to half a mile wide. Within the city, an area 4 blocks wide and 8 miles long was totally destroyed. 633 homes were destroyed, 12 people were killed, and there were 2 further deaths from heart disease. 70 people were admitted to

hospital and 316 treated as outpatients. Exceptionally good warning was given by radio and TV announcements 15–20 min before the impact.

(5) Wichita Falls: 6.15 p.m. April 10, 1979 [24]. This was rated at 4 on the Fujita scale[6] of tornado strength, placing it in the severest 3% of tornadoes in the United States. 3,000 homes were destroyed or rendered uninhabitable as the tornado tracked across the city. 47 people were killed and hundreds more injured.

Aspects Relating to Death and Injury. Published observations on these tornado incidents provide some information on four aspects relating to death and injury: (1) the location of people killed and injured at the time of impact; (2) cause of death; (3) types of injury; and (4) some age- and sex-specific data.

(1) Location of People at Time of Impact. The damage caused by a tornado is dramatic but confined to a clearly defined area. Only one paper [6] gives details of the location of the dead and injured in relation to the area of destruction; in the Topeka tornado, it was found that all deaths occurred within the main tornado track and all serious injuries in only a slightly wider band.

Information on the specific location of people killed and injured within a tornado area is more plentiful. This question is of interest because of its relevance to advice and warnings given to the residents of tornado-prone areas. Of the 17 people killed in the Lebanon, Ind. tornado of 1965, 10 had been at home, and 7 were riding in motorcars. Of the 24 patients admitted to hospital, 20 had been at home; in many instances, the house had been blown away, and the patient was found some yards away. 4 patients admitted to hospital were riding in cars at the time of the storm, and in all instances the car was lifted into the air and thrown across fields [46]. 1 of the patients died in a hospital admitting room. While 3 who had been in cars survived, 'most of their fellow passengers died immediately of severe cerebro-cranial trauma' [46].

The Wichita falls tornado caused 43 traumatic deaths and 59 serious injuries. 26 of the deaths (60%) and 30 of the serious injuries (51%) occurred to the occupants of cars [24]. Only 5 people were killed at home at the time of the strike. 'Of the 59 people injured in their vehicles, 43

---

[6] The Fujita scale ranks tornado damage from 0–5. Strength 4 corresponds to a maximum wind velocity of 335 km/h [74].

Table III. Causes of death in the Indiana and Topeka tornadoes

Topeka		Lebanon, Ind.	
Head and chest injuries	4	skull and brain injury	14
Chest injuries	4	'crushed chest trauma'	2
Head injuries	2	cervical spine fracture and cord injury	1
Massive trauma to body	1		
Shock, abrasions and lacerations	1		
Total	12		17

Data from *Beelman* [6] and *Mandelbaum* et al. [46].

(73%) had entered their vehicles expressly to outrun the tornado. The homes left by 20 of these victims, including 8 of those who died, suffered little or no damage according to a Red Cross housing survey . . .' In Wichita Falls, people in mobile homes appeared to be at most risk, although only four serious injuries and no deaths occurred in this group. *Glass* [24] calculated the relative risk of death or serious injury in various groups to be 3:1,000 in people who remained in stationary homes, 23:1,000 in cars and 85:1,000 in mobile homes.

(2) Causes of Death. Of the five studies of tornado strike, two give some information on cause of death. In Worcester, several people were decapitated, and many suffered a severe crushing injury of the skull [4]. Among the latter, several were observed with an empty cranium, and it is thought that the cranial contents had been sucked out completely by the wind. Crushing wounds of the chest and trunk were also reported in 2 or 3 patients who died soon after injury. In Indiana, it was noted that severe cerebro-cranial trauma accounted for 14 of the 17 immediate deaths in the county, which *Mandelbaum* et al. [46] attributed to both the particular risks of motorcars and to injuries sustained from high-velocity flying objects. A relatively large proportion of deaths seen in Topeka were also from head and chest injuries (see table III).

(3) Types of Injury. The types of injuries seen in hospitalised casualties in each of the tornadoes show a broad similarity (see Table IV). There is a high proportion of head injury including skull fracture, other fractures, lacerations and abrasions. Severe and extensive soft tissue injury was noted in Indiana in all patients. A large proportion of heavily contaminated wounds has been noted in tornado casualties. 'In most instances, foreign

Table IV. Percent of serious injuries noted following three tornadoes

	Worcester[1]	Dallas[2]	Wichita Falls[3]
Fractures			
Skull (including severe head and cerebral injury)	17.0	21.9	14.3/7.8[4]
Upper extremity	10.2	–	16.1/13.6
Lower extremity	9.3	–	21.4/15.5
Ribs	7.1	–	19.6/11.7
Shoulder girdle	4.6	–	–
Pelvis	2.2	–	3.6/2.9
Hip	1.1	–	–
Nose	0.9	–	–
Cervical spine	0.7	–	–
Back injury including fracture	3.3	–	8.9/5.8[5]
Jaw	0.4	–	–
Other sites	–	43.7	1.8/1.9
N	257	21	48/33
Other injuries			
Eye	6.2	–	–
Kidney	2.0	–	–
Spleen	1.3	–	–
Burns	1.1	–	–
Major lacerations, contusions, soft tissue trauma	32.6	28.1	14.3/40.8
Shock	+[6]	–	–
Chest injury	–[7]	6.3	–
Traumatic amputation	+	–	–
N	195	11	8/23

Data obtained from *Bakst* et al. [4], *Fogelman* [20] and *Glass* et al. [24].
[1] Worcester: 452 injuries noted in 438 patients. Data probably refer to patients admitted to hospital.
[2] Dallas: data refer to 32 patients of 74 admitted to Park Memorial hospital.
[3] Wichita Falls: patients admitted to hospital and retained for at least 1 week.
[4] First figure refers to primary diagnosis on admission to hospital, second figure to secondary diagnosis.
[5] Classified as vertebral fractures.
[6] Injury noted to have occurred.
[7] Category is not applicable.

materials such as splinters, tar, dirt and manure were embedded deeply into areas of soft tissue injury' [46]. In Worcester, a similar pattern of wound contamination was noted in many patients [30]: 'Some of the casualties exhibited extensive deep abrasions due to the sand-blast effect of dirt and debris striking at high velocity. The clothing in such cases was torn off by the force of the blast'. In Topeka, casualties were said to be 'typical of tornado victims: dirty, wet with torn clothing, cuts, abrasions, bruises . . .' [6].

The contamination of wounds appears to be a major contributing factor to a high rate of post-operative sepsis, even under conditions where casualties received highly skilled and prompt surgical debridement. In Worcester [4], the authors made a determined effort to estimate the wound sepsis rate. They found that sepsis was frequent in both minor and major injuries. Estimates of sepsis rates in minor wounds varied from one-half to two-thirds of all cases. On July 27, 1953, almost 7 weeks after the tornado, 612 victims were still being treated in their homes, mostly for septic wounds. *Hight* et al. [30] examined the post-operative course of patients after the Worcester tornado and found sepsis in 12.5–23.0% of orthopaedic and neurosurgical patients with lacerations. In addition, 3 cases of gas gangrene were noted and no cases of tetanus. No cases of gas gangrene were reported in the Indiana series [46]. One case of tetanus was seen in an elderly woman after the Wichita Falls tornado [24].

Two studies have looked specifically at the causes of bacterial contamination of wounds sustained during tornadoes. After the Lubbock tornado, which occurred at 9.30 a.m. on May 11, 1970, bacteriological studies of wounds conducted by *Gilbert* et al. [22] revealed frequent infection with aerobic gram-negative bacilli, attributed to intense soil contamination. The degree of force of contamination is well illustrated by 1 patient in Lubbock who 'was still coughing up grass 4 days after injury'. After the tornado of April 11, 1965, in Elkhart county, Indiana, *Ivy* [34] compared the frequency and types of infection in tornado victims with a control group of motorcar accident victims. He found the frequency of infection to be much higher in the tornado victims, with a slightly (though not significantly) higher incidence of infections arising from enterobacteria.

(4) Age- and Sex-Specific Data. In Wichita Falls, age- and sex-specific rates of fatal and serious non-fatal injury were calculated [24]. Rates were found to increase with age. People over age 60 were injured seven times more frequently than individuals under age 20. Above the age of 40 years, women were at greater risk of injury than men, and above the age of 60 years, this

difference was almost twofold. Of the 12 tornado deaths in Topeka [6], 9 were males and 3 were females. No information is available on the sex of the seriously injured. Of the 9 males, 7 were age 59 or over; the 3 females were all over age 90. The 24 people hospitalised after the Indiana tornado were equally divided between males and females. The age range was from 4 to 80 years, although 8 were between 70 and 80 years [46].

The three accounts, therefore, suggest that the risk increases with age but may vary by sex. The accounts of the tornadoes do not indicate why this should be so, but it is presumably due to differences in car, house and mobile home occupancy at the time the tornado struck.

Variations in Tornado Risk within Continental United States. Tornado mortality in the southern United States is much higher than in the rest of the USA. *Sims and Baumann* [59] have shown that this is not due to a greater frequency or severity of tornadoes in these areas, to a greater frequency of nocturnal strikes, or to a better warning system. Differences in building styles in the areas suggest that risk should be the reverse of that actually observed. The wood-framed buildings generally used in the south appear, because of better ventilation and faster pressure equilibration, to resist destruction, or to collapse piecemeal, whereas the masonry buildings used in the north collapse as a unit. *Sims and Baumann* suggest, on the basis of a survey of attitudes, that the difference in mortality may be due, at least in part, to response to warnings. Southerners show a 'much higher degree of fatalism, possibly lack of trust in and inattention to warning systems'.

Cyclonic Storm Surge, Tsunami and Other Floods

Floods are the commonest of all natural disasters and cause greater mortality than any other type of disaster. Almost every country is prone to floods. A rough calculation based on an analysis of a series of large, natural disasters suggests that floods (including storm surge) account for approximately 50% of disasters and a similar proportion of deaths [17].

Floods may occur for many reasons, and for the topic of this chapter, no completely satisfactory classification is possible. In general terms, floods arise from: (1) the over-topping of rivers; (2) rainfall and snow; (3) the rupture of dams and glacial lakes; and (4) cyclonic storm surge and tsunami.

However, given the worldwide incidence of floods and the vast range of conditions in different areas, these categories are of only limited use. In considering total mortality, the major division appears to be between the first two categories, where escape is often possible and mortality generally low; and the last two categories where, in densely populated areas, many thousands may die. From the perspective of this section, the point is of almost academic interest as the relevant literature is very small. To some extent this may reflect the fact, as with wind disaster, that floods of any type appear to cause few injuries of any severity in survivors. Many accounts of specific floods mention total mortality, but either do not mention or, more rarely, exclude a specific problem arising from injuries in survivors. The storm surge and tsunami have specific characteristics which are described here.

The Cyclonic Storm Surge

This is caused partly by the pressure differential within a cyclonic storm (see cyclone, p. 00) and partly by high winds acting directly on the water. This results in a mass of water above the general sea level moving at the same speed as the cyclone (possibly only 10 mph or so). The effect of this mass of water striking a coastline depends upon a number of factors: the forward speed of the cyclone; the angle of the sea bed; the funnelling effects of bays and estuaries; and perhaps most important, the height of the tide. Waves riding on top of the surge may also cause damage. After striking the coast a storm surge will move inland, often at considerable speed, and will only be stopped by high land. Although the water will then begin to retreat, it may be retained by the high wind, and persist until the 'eye' of the storm has passed, a period of perhaps 3–5 h.

Of all areas of the world, the countries bordering the Indian ocean and particularly those bordering the Bay of Bengal, have suffered most from cyclones and sea surges. In the northern Bay of Bengal, a unique combination of high tides, a 'funnelling' coastal configuation, low flat terrain and a high population density have produced some of the largest mortality figures associated with any type of disaster. 13 out of 19 'noteworthy' tropical cyclone disasters listed by *Frank and Hussein* [21] over a 250-year period, occurred in India or East Pakistan. In the same period the western hemisphere has suffered only three comparable events. In the period 1960–1970, East Pakistan (Bangladesh) alone lost an average of 5,000 people/year to this cause, excluding the mortality from the great 1970 cyclone and storm surge.

The East Bengal Cyclone of November 1970. This cyclone, and a massive, accompanying tidal bore struck the southern coastal region of East Pakistan (now Bangladesh) on November 12/13. The cyclone affected approximately 650 square miles, about half of which was directly affected by the storm surge. The population density of the area was approximately 330 people per square km, made up largely of farmers (80%) and fishermen (12%). Most cyclones originate in the Bay of Bengal in spring and summer; the unseasonal timing of this cyclone compounded the tragedy by striking when the crop was being harvested and 100,000 labourers were living in the fields. Houses in the area are built mainly of jute stalks and bamboo, usually with only one room, and are roofed with straw or rarely with corrugated iron.

Two surveys were conducted by *Sommer and Mosely* [60] after the cyclone: The first, between November 28 and December 2, concerned immediate medical needs and water supply; and the second, between February 10 and March 4, 1971, compiled information for long-term relief and recovery. These surveys were carefully designed and can be considered to be representative of the population affected.

Death and Injury. In the first survey, mortality was estimated at 240,000, 14.2% of the population. Cyclone-related morbidity was largely limited to minor cuts and bruises and an occasional fracture, although one clinical entity dubbed 'cyclone syndrome' was quite common. This syndrome consisted of severe abrasions of the arms, chest and thighs, testifying to the tenacity with which survivors clung to trees to withstand the buffeting of the tidal bore. In the second survey, a larger sample was taken (3,000 families, 1.4% of the affected population) and more detailed enquiries were made. Mortality was found to vary mainly with distance from the coast. In one inland area, mortality was estimated at 4.7%, rising to 46.3% in a severely affected coastal union (the smallest administrative subdivision). On many offshore islands, entire populations died. It is also reported that of 77,000 inshore fishermen operating in the affected area, 46,000 lost their lives [21].

Age- and Sex-Specific Mortality. More than half of all deaths were found to be of children under 10 years of age, a group representing only ⅓ of the population. Mortality was also much higher in people over 50 years of age. Males fared better than females in all but the youngest age groups. The highest survival rates were of adult males between the ages of

15 and 45 years, consistent with the impression that 'those too weak to cling to trees, the old, young, sick and malnourished, and females in general, were selectively lost in the storm'. These mortality figures are similar to the pattern seen after some earthquakes (see fig. 7).

The Andhra Pradesh Cyclone and Storm Surge

On the night of November 19/20, 1977, a cyclone, heavy rainfall and a storm surge struck part of coastal Andhra Pradesh in southeast India. Although a long stretch of coast was affected, the delta of the Krishna river caught the worst of the wave. Along the front of the river delta, the wave was 15 ft high, reducing to 3 ft further inland. The wave moved at about 10 mph and penetrated inland for 10 miles. Together, the cyclone and storm surge affected an area of approximately 7,500 square miles. Approximately 400 mm of rain fell in a 6 to 7-hour period.

The quality of data available on this disaster is poorer than that on the East Bengal cyclone; even so, a very similar pattern of death and injury is found. A total of 710,000 people in 2,302 villages was reported to have been affected by the storm surge and/or the cyclone and torrential rain; 8,504 killed and 3,000 missing [16]. Of those killed, 6,734 died in Krishna district and 1,519 in Guntur. In seven adjacent districts, only 68 people were killed [16]. Within Krishna district the great majority of deaths occurred within the area affected by the storm surge. *Cohen and Raghavulu* [14] gave a different estimate of mortality within Krishna district (8,033), but reported that of these, 6,892 died in the storm surge area. The great majority of deaths in this district occurred in Devi, a headland at the mouth of the river. Even within Devi, there was wide variation in reported mortality (range 0–81.9% of the pre-cyclone population): of 33 villages for which data are available, 5 (15%) lost more than 50% of their population, and in 18 (55%), more than 10% died [14].

Most of the 1,519 people reported killed in Guntur are reported to have died as a result of building collapse due to the high winds and torrential rain [16].

Of the 6,892 killed in the storm surge area of Krishna district, 1,291 were reported to be adult males, 1,944 adult females, and 3,657 children. Although these groups are not specified exactly, this suggests a pattern of mortality similar to that in Bengal in 1970 [14].

Injuries in survivors were due mainly to the collapse of buildings and flying debris. Orthopaedic cases numbered 177. These were mainly fractures of the extremities, evacuated to a government hospital. There were

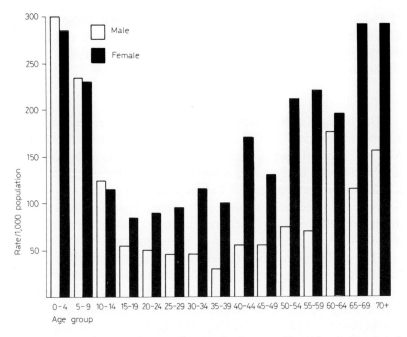

Fig. 7. Age- and sex-specific mortality rates in the area affected by the Bangladesh cyclone and storm surge of November 1970. Figures for males based on 1,359 enumerated deaths; figures for females on 1,583 enumerated deaths. Data from published graph by *Sommer and Mosley* [60].

5 cases of spinal injury and paraplegia, and 16 died in hospital from multiple injuries [16]. Minor surgical cases consisted mainly of lacerations and penetrating wounds of the feet from walking on thorns. According to *Winchester* [77], most of the injuries were minor cuts and bruises, and many victims were suffering from shock and exposure, indicating a greater need for paramedical personnel than for doctors.

Tsunami and Other Floods

The tsunami results from sudden movements of the seabed mostly caused by undersea earthquakes. These movements displace large volumes of water, causing a wave of low amplitude but long wavelength, which travels at a speed roughly proportional to the square root of the depth of the water. In the deep oceans, the wave may travel at speeds up to 750 km/h. As it reaches coastal and shallower waters, the amplitude of the wave increases and may reach heights of 20 m or more in bays, where a funnelling effect occurs. Damage and loss of life may occur at great distances from the point of origin of the wave. For example, the tsunami set up by the Chilean earthquake of 1960 caused 61 deaths in Hawaii [2].

The tsunami hazard for all practical purposes is confined to the countries which border the Pacific ocean, although they have occurred rarely in the Atlantic. Perhaps the best known example is the tsunami which was set up by the Lisbon earthquake of 1755, which caused great tides as far away as Barbados and floods in Norway and Germany [74].

We have found no detailed accounts of mortality and injury resulting from tsunami, although there are many reports of total deaths in specific incidents. The tsunami resulting from the Krakatoa volcanic explosion in 1883 is said to have drowned some 36,000 people in Sumatra and Java [2]. In 1896, 27,000 people died in Java from a tsunami after the Sanriki earthquake in Japan. More recently, in 1976 a 20 ft tsunami was reported to have killed 'thousands' in Mindenaio in the Philippines, virtually wiping out some villages [45]. *Haas* [28] reports that there were an estimated 5,820 dead and missing in this tsunami, of whom 85% were victims of the waves, which penetrated inland to a depth of up to half a mile. In the United States, however, where reasonably accurate statistics are available, casualties from tsunami have amounted to only approximately 396 killed and 640 'injured' during the period between 1906 and 1965.

From the physical nature of a tsunami, it might be supposed that its effects would be much the same as those of a major dam burst. That is, the absolute mortality would be a function of the size and other characteristics of the tsunami, as well as the population of the affected area, but there would be a few serious injuries in survivors.

The Vaiont Dam Overflow. At 10.40 p.m. on October 9, 1963, an enormous landslide, estimated at between 200 and 400 million cubic metres fell into the lake behind the Vaiont dam in north Italy. Over 100 million tons of water were displaced over the dam top and crashed into the Piave River Valley, almost obliterating the town of Longorone and several nearby hamlets. In Longorone itself, 1,269 out of 1,348 people known to be in the town were killed, and an additional 727 persons were killed in nearby locations.

Quarentelli [56], drawing on a study by the Disaster Research Group reports that there was 'an extremely high ratio of killed to injured, probably in the range of 40 dead for every non-fatal casualty. Even in absolute terms there were only 60–80 injured.' He also notes that this had interesting consequences for the relief operation: 'Organisations at a distance, and distant higher headquarters of organisations operating in the impact area kept inquiring why the groups on the scene did not request medical supplies, physicians, blankets, etc. Working with the usual image of disasters where there are always more injured than dead, they found it difficult to comprehend that in this catastrophe there were almost no survivors.'

Following repeated requests from outside as to why these types of assistance were not being requested, some 'officials on the scene almost seemed to feel that they were being accused of dereliction of their responsibilities because they did not make such requests'.

Rapid City, South Dakota. On June 9, 1972, torrential rain caused flooding and heavy damage along the course of the Rapid Creek which runs through Rapid City. Just before midnight, a dam gave way, sending a 5 ft wall of water along the course of the creek, killing 238 people. 'Accurate figures for the number and types of injuries are not available. It should be pointed out that this particular disaster did not cause a large number of severe injuries. With the exception of three or four burns and a lesser number of fractures, most of the patients were treated for lacerations, abrasions and exposure. At St. John's hospital, 77 patients were admitted and 330 seen in the emergency room in the 48 hours following the flood' [15]. The bed occupancy of St. John's hospital, even allowing for transfers from another flooded hospital, did not exceed 90% [19].

The Netherlands Flood. The Netherlands flood of February 1, 1953, resulting from the breach of a polder, affected extensive areas of the country and caused 1,795 deaths, mainly through drowning. Six medical problems were identified after the flood [3]: (1) identifying and recovering corpses; (2) evacuating the sick and old; (3) providing physicians with routine supplies; (4) setting up emergency hospitals to take care of the evacuated; (5) restoring hygienic services, and (6) taking measures to fight epidemics. It was explicitly stated that the injured, as a group, did not represent a medical problem.

The age- and sex-specific mortality of those killed in the flood is shown in figure 8. It should be noted that the rates were calculated using a population which may not be exactly representative of the population in the flooded area.

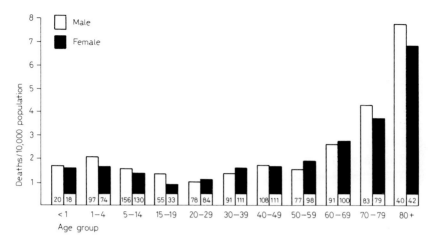

Fig. 8. Age- and sex-specific mortality in the February 1, 1953 Netherlands flood. Numbers in bars represent absolute numbers of deaths. Data from *Baesjou* [3]. Calculated using population data for December 31, 1952, from Statistical Yearbook of the Netherlands 1953–1954, Netherlands Central Bureau of Statistics.

The Bristol Flood, England: July 10/11, 1968. On July 10/11 1968, between 5 a.m. and 5 p.m., 13 cm of rain fell on the city of Bristol in western England. About 3,000 houses, shops and other buildings were flooded. Many other areas of southwestern England were also affected, but Bristol was particularly hard hit as the tidal river Avon runs through its centre. The peak of the rainfall coincided with a high spring tide which blocked the outflow into the river. The water level reached no higher than the ceilings of the ground floor and subsided, in most cases, after about 10 h, leaving a fine layer of stinking mud. One man was drowned in the flood.

Bennet [8] investigated mortality, general practitioner attendance, referral to hospital and hospital admission for the occupants of 88 houses which had been flooded (population = 316) and a control group of 132 houses which had not (population = 434), for the 12-month period before and after the flood. He found that surgery attendance of the flooded population for whom records were available (66% of the flooded group, 52% not flooded) increased by 53% (males 81%, females 25%) although the total number of people attending did not change substantially. The non-flooded group showed a slight fall in attendance. The difference between the attendance for flooded and non-flooded men was statistically significant (p < 0.001) as was the difference in the attendance within the flooded group for the period before and after the flood. The increase in attendance by women was not significant. Hospital referrals from the flooded group more than doubled during the year after the flood. This was again accounted for mainly by men. Hospital admissions showed the same trend.

The reasons for admission 'read almost as though they were a random selection'. These included arterial insufficiency, injury unrelated to the flood and routine surgery, but no diagnosis which suggested any direct physical relationship with the flood.

Mortality rates were also calculated for all homes in the city and county of Bristol which had been flooded on July 10/11, 1968, as well as those which had not been flooded. The number of deaths from the flooded addresses for the 12-month period before and the 12-month period after the floods was compared with the rest (non-flooded area) of the city. Surprisingly, mortality in the flooded group increased by 50%, from 58 deaths in the year before the flood to 87 deaths in the following year. The most pronounced rise was in the age group 45–64 where male deaths increased from 7 to 20 and female deaths from 5 to 9. These occurred mainly in the third 3-month period after the flood. Otherwise the increases were predominantly amongst those over 65, especially women over age 75 (from 9 deaths pre-flood to 19 after). For the rest of Bristol (non-flooded), deaths fell by 1%. The increased mortality in the flooded group was significant (p < 0.02).

Cause of death was established from death certificates, but only diagnoses of specific malignant diseases were felt to be sufficiently reliable to enable making accurate pre- and post-flood comparisons. In the flooded group there were 9 deaths from malignant disease; in the year after, there were 21. For the rest of Bristol (non-flooded) the deaths from malignant disease over the same periods were 1,010 and 1,060, respectively. The difference between the flooded and non-flooded groups just failed to reach a level of significance.

Bennet [8] could find no direct physical cause for the increase in mortality either related or unrelated to the flood. He attempted to explain the observation in terms of the psychological effects of the flooding.

Lorraine [44] described a similar pattern of mortality in Canvey Island, southeastern England, after floods in 1953.

Secondary Disasters

The popular notion that earthquakes and other disasters are followed in quick succession by firestorm, breach of dams, tidal waves and the like, seems only rarely to have been fulfilled in reality. After a natural disaster has struck, there are two main risks to survivors. First, from true 'secondary' disaster which is triggered off by the primary event, e.g. breach of a dam. This appears to have occurred only after earthquakes, and then only rarely. Second, there is the much more regular, but generally minor risk of physical injury faced by survivors in the altered post-disaster environment.

Fire

Both the Tokyo earthquake of 1923 and the 1906 San Francisco earthquake were followed by major fires. In Tokyo, it is probable that fire resulted in more casualties than the earthquake itself [74]. The densely packed and highly inflammable buildings were engulfed in a firestorm which destroyed some three-quarters of Tokyo/Yokohama. In more recent earthquakes, fire has rarely occurred. This is presumably because the areas struck were those in which mud or rock was the primary building material used, or areas where minor fires could be easily extinguished, such as San Fernando. In San Fernando, burns made up 7% of all out-patients seen after the 1971 earthquake [53]. *Whittaker* et al. [76] note that some patients were treated for burns after the 1972 Managua earthquake, but it is clear from other accounts that there was no major conflagration.

Avalanche

The 1970 Peruvian earthquake triggered a massive avalanche from Mount Huascaran (6,665 m) in which a huge block of ice and rock approximately 800 by 300 m fell from the mountain. The avalanche of debris it set in motion travelled a horizontal distance of 16 km in just under 2 min, obliterating 10 small villages, part of the town of Ranrahirca and practically the whole town of Yungay [13].

It is, of course, possible that a considerable range of other secondary disasters could follow earthquakes: the Vaiont Dam overflow washed away eight large drums of potassium cyanide from a local factory [56] although they were recovered intact. The risks to nuclear power plants from earthquakes are potentially very serious, and many other risks 'secondary' to earthquake might be imagined.

Other Risks

Few authors mention deaths or injuries in survivors of events secondary to earthquakes or other natural catastrophes. *Whittaker* et al.[76] notes two specific problems after the Managua earthquake: first, injuries resulting from automobile and motorcycle accidents increased after the earthquake; and, second, the trauma of social chaos as the 'pistol and machete replaced established legal procedures'. Numerous patients were treated for wounds.[7] Deaths have also occurred in people searching through damaged buildings [29] and penetrating wounds of the feet have been noted after several types of disaster [16, 27]. This does not, however, appear to have amounted to a significant medical problem.

Conclusions

Several conclusions appear to be justified even from the limited evidence presented in this chapter. Although the case examples are few, the relationship between the physical effects of each disaster type, and the observed pattern of death and injury is sufficiently direct that even if the conclusions cannot be accepted as 'rules', at least they may be expected to apply in many parts of the world.

(1) The effect of disasters in terms of both the absolute and relative numbers of people killed and injured is related to the disaster type. After earthquakes, cyclones and tornadoes, traumatic injuries are likely to exceed the number of deaths, often by a factor of two or three. Deaths are likely to exceed the number of injuries caused by all types of flood, including cyclonic storm surge. The absolute number of serious injuries is likely to be large (i.e. in the thousands) only after major earthquakes. The number of serious injuries caused by all types of floods, cyclones and tornadoes is likely to be, relative to earthquakes, small.

(2) After earthquakes, minor injuries (i.e. not requiring hospital admission) are likely to outnumber serious injuries by as many as 10:1.

(3) The pattern of injury observed appears to be relatively specific to the type of disaster, even among different countries. In the case of tornadoes, at least in the USA, the pattern of injury is very specific.

---

[7] This pattern of behaviour appears to be very rare following natural disasters [18] and may have been related to the political circumstances in the country at that time.

(4) With the rare exception of earthquakes followed by a major confla-gration, the overwhelming majority of injuries are sustained during the main disaster impact. The period of need for emergency services varies with the size of the affected area and the communications therein. It is likely to be confined to the first week post-impact, and concentrated in the first 3–5 days.

(5) Death and injury occur differentially in various age and sex groups, tending to favour the survival of adults in the most economically active age groups, particularly the survival of adult men.

References

1   Altay, F.: Disasters in Turkey. Joint IHF/IUA/UNDRO/WHO Seminar, Manila 1978.
2   Ayre, R.S.; Mileti, D.S.: Earthquake and tsunami hazards in the United States – a re-search assessment (Institute of Behavioral Science, Boulder 1975).
3   Baesjou, J.F.: Problems of medicine during and after the flood in the Netherlands. Wld med. J. 2: 351–353 (1955).
4   Bakst, H.J.; Berg, R.L.; Foster, F.D.; Raker, J.W.: The Worcester County tornado. A medical study of the disaster. Committee on Disaster Studies (National Research Council, Washington 1954).
5   Bay Area Earthquake Response Planning Project: Estimates from: Steinbrugge, Alger-missen, A study of earthquake losses in the San Francisco Bay area (US Department of Commerce/National Oceanic and Atmospheric Administration Environmental Re-search Laboratories, 1972), and An analysis of 'a study of earthquake losses in the San Francisco Bay area' disaster preparedness (Office of Emergency Preparedness, Executive Office of the President, 1972); in Earthquake data file (The Open University, Milton Keynes 1976).
6   Beelman, F.C.: Disaster planning, report of tornado casualties in Topeka. J. Kans. med. Soc. 68: 153–161 (1967).
7   Beinin, L.: An examination of health data following two Russian earthquakes. Disasters 5: 142–146 (1981).
8   Bennet, G.: Bristol flood 1968 – controlled survey of effects on health of local commu-nity disaster. Br. med. J. iii: 454–458 (1970).
9   Berberian, M.: Tabas-E-Golshan (Iran) – catastrophic earthquake of Sept. 16 1978: a preliminary field report. Disasters 2: 207–219 (1978).
10   Berg, G.: The Skopje Yugoslavia earthquake, July 26, 1963 (American Iron & Steel Institute, New York 1964).
11   Berlin, G.L.: Earthquakes and the urban environment, vol. I (CRC Press, Boca Raton 1980).
12   Bywaters, E.G.L.: Ischaemic muscle necrosis. J. Am. med. Ass. 124: 1103–1107 (1944).
13   Clapperton, C.M.: Volcanic and earthquake disasters. British Association for the Advancement of Science, Leicester 1972.
14   Cohen, S.P.; Raghavulu, C.V.: The Andhra cyclone of 1977 (Vikas, New Delhi 1979).

15   Coolidge, T.T.: Rapid City flood medical response. Archs Surg., Chicago *106:* 770–772 (1973).

16   Dharmaraju, P.: Emergency health and medical care in cyclone and tidal wave affected areas of Andhra Pradesh. Joint IHF/IUA/UNDRO/WHO Seminar, Manila 1978.

17   Dworkin, J.: Global trends in natural disasters, 1947–1973. Natural Hazards Working Paper No. 26 (University of Colorado, Boulder, undated).

18   Dynes, R.R.; Quarentelli, E.L.; Kreps, G.A.: A perspective on disaster planning. Disaster Research Series No. 11 (Ohio State University, Columbus 1972).

19   Flood disaster, Rapid City, South Dakota (Public Health Service-HSM-CDC, Atlanta 1972).

20   Fogelman, M.J.: The Dallas tornado disaster. Am. J. Surg. *95:* 501–507 (1958).

21   Frank, N.L.; Hussein, S.A.: The deadliest tropical cyclone in history? Bull. Am. met. Soc. *52:* 438–444 (1971).

22   Gilbert, D.N.; Sandford, J.P.; Kutscher, E.; Sanders, C.V.; Luby, J.P.; Barnett, J.A.: Microbiologic study of wound infections in tornado casualties. Archs envir. Hlth *26:* 125–130 (1973).

23   Glass, R.I.; Urrutia, J.J.; Sibornys, S.; Smith, H.: Earthquake injuries related to housing in a Guatemalan village. Science, N.Y. *197:* 638–643 (1977).

24   Glass, R.I.; Craven, R.B.; Bregman, D.J.; Stoll, B.J.; Horowitz, N.; Kerndt, P.; Winkle, J.: Injuries from the Wichita Falls tornado – implications for prevention. Science, N.Y. *207:* 734–738 (1980).

25   Goll, F.: Die Erdbeben Chiles. Münch. geog. Stud. *14:* 93 (1904).

26   Gouin, P.: Earthquake history of Ethiopia and the Horn of Africa (International Development Research Centre, Ottawa 1979).

27   Gurd, C.H.; Bromwich, A.; Quinn, J.V.: Health management of cyclone Tracy. Med. J. Aust. *i:* 641–644 (1975).

28   Haas, J.E.: The Philippine earthquake and tsunami disaster – a reexamination of some behavioral propositions. Disasters *2:* 3–9 (1978).

29   Haas, J.E.: The Western Sicily earthquake of 1968 (National Academy of Sciences, Washington 1969).

30   Hight, D.; Blodgett, J.T.; Croce, E.J.; Horne, E.O.; McKoan, J.W.; Whelan, C.S.: Medical aspects of the Worcester tornado disaster. New Engl. J. Med. *254:* 267–271 (1956).

31   Hogg, S.J.: Reconstruction following seismic disaster in Venzone Friuli. Disasters *4:* 173–186 (1980).

32   Iacopi, R.: Earthquake country (Lane Book Co., California 1964); cited in *Nichols* [52].

33   Ilhan, E.: Earthquakes in Turkey; in Geology and history of Turkey. Petrol.Explor.Soc. Libya, Annu. Field Conf. No 13, (1971), pp. 431–442.

34   Ivy, J.H.: Infections encountered in tornado and automobile accident victims. J. Ind. St. med. Ass. *61:* 1657–1661 (1968).

35   James, P.: Catch the wind. The Guardian (London 30.7.81).

36   Kates, R.W.; Haas, J.E.; Amarel, D.J.; Olson, R.A.; Ramos, R.; Olson, R.: Human impact of the Managua earthquake. Science, N.Y. *182:* 981–990 (1973).

37   League of Red Cross Societies: Bangladesh tornado. Relief Bureau Circular No. 823 (League of Red Cross Societies, Geneva 1981).

38   Leimena, S.L.: Traditional Balinese earthquake-proof housing structures. Disasters *4:* 247–250 (1980).

39   Leimena, S.L.: Disaster in Bali caused by earthquake. A report. Disasters *3:* 85–87
      (1979).

40   Lomnitz, C.: Casualties and behaviour of populations during earthquakes. Bull. Am.
      seism. Soc. *60:* 1309–1313 (1970).

41   London Technical Group: The Lice earthquake – a briefing document (London Tech-
      nical Group, London 1975).

42   Long, E.C.: The dilemmas of disaster – some medical aspects of the Guatemala earth-
      quake (Rockefeller Foundation, New York, undated).

43   Long, E.C.: Sermons in stones – some medical aspects of the earthquake in Guatemala.
      St. Mary's Hospital Gazette, LXXXIII, 2; pp. 6–9 (London 1977).

44   Lorraine, N.S.W.: Cited in *Bennet* [8].

45   Majarocon, V.P.: The Mindenao earthquake/tsunami disaster. Joint IHF/IUA/
      UNDRO/WHO Seminar, Manila 1978.

46   Mandelbaum, I.; Nahrwold, D.; Boyer, D.W.: Management of tornado casualties. J.
      Trauma *6:* 353–367 (1966).

47   Manning, D.H.: Disaster technology – an annotated bibliography (Pergamon Press,
      Oxford 1973).

48   Memarzadeh, P.: The earthquake of August 31 1968 in the south of Khorasan, Iran.
      Joint IHF/IUA/UNDRO/WHO Seminar, Manila 1978.

49   Milne, G.: Cyclone Tracy. I. Some consequences of evacuation for adult victims. Aust.
      Psychol. *12:* 39–49 (1977).

50   Mirouze, J.: Etude clinique des nephropathies par ensevelissment du seisme d'Agadir,
      du 1er Mars 1960. Maroc med. *40:* 137–149 (1961).

51   Mitchell, W.A.: Reconstruction after disaster. The Gediz earthquake of 1970. Geograph.
      Rev. *66:* 296–313 (1976).

52   Nichols, T.C.: Global summary of human response to natural hazards: earthquakes; in
      Disaster data file, pp. 6–14 (The Open University, Milton Keynes 1976).

53   Olsen, R.A.: Individual and organizational dimensions of the San Francisco earthquake;
      in Berjer, Coffman, Dees, San Fernando California earthquake of Feb. 9 1971. (US
      Department of Commerce, Washington 1973).

54   Peavy, J.G.: Hurricane Beulah. Am. J. publ. Hlth *60:* 481–484 (1970).

55   Populazione e movimento anagrafico dei communi (Instituto Centrale di Statistica,
      Rome 1977).

56   Quarentelli, E.L.: The Vaiont Dam overflow – a case study of extracommunity responses
      in massive disasters. Disasters *3:* 199–212 (1979).

57   Romero, A.B.; Cobar, R.; Western, K.A.; Lopez, S.M.: Some epidemiological features
      of disasters in Guatemala. Disasters *2:* 39–46 (1978).

58   Saidi, F.: The 1962 earthquake in Iran – some medical and social aspects. New Engl. J.
      Med. *268:* 929–932 (1963).

59   Sims, D.D.; Baumann, J.H.: The tornado threat – coping styles of the north and south.
      Science, N.Y. *176:* 1386–1392 (1972).

60   Sommer, A.; Mosely, W.H.: East Bengal cyclone of November 1970 – epidemiological
      approach to disaster assessment. Lancet *i:* 1029–1036 (1972).

61   Sri Lanka Cyclone Handbook: Sri Lanka cyclone study technical report No. 7 (PADCO
      Inc., Washington 1979).

62   Steinbrugge, K.V.; Cluff, L.S.: The Caracas Venezuela earthquake of July 29 1967.
      Mineral Information Service, vol. 21, pp. 3–13; cited in *Nichols* [52].

63 Stephenson, R.: Personal commun.

64 United Nations Disaster Relief Coordinator: Report on the cyclone and torrential rains in the Sultanate of Oman, June 1977 (UNDRO, Geneva 1977).

65 United Nations Disaster Relief Coordinator: Disaster prevention and mitigation, a compendium of current knowledge, vol. 4. Meteorological aspects (United Nations, New York 1978).

66 United Nations Disaster Relief Coordinator: Report on the cyclone in Sri Lanka, November 23/24 1978 (UNDRO, Geneva 1979).

67 United Nations Disaster Relief Coordinator: Report on hurricane David in Dominica, August 29, 1979 (UNDRO, Geneva 1980).

68 United Nations Disaster Relief Coordinator: Report on hurricanes David and Frederick in the Dominican Republic, August/September 1979 (UNDRO, Geneva 1980).

69 Ville de Goyet, C. de; Lechat, M.; Boucquey, C.: Drugs and supplies for disaster relief. Trop. Doctor 6: 168–170 (1976).

70 Ville de Goyet, C. de; Cid, E. del; Romero, A.; Jeannée, E.; Lechat, M.: Earthquake in Guatemala – epidemiologic evaluation of the relief effort. Bull. Pan Am. Hlth Org. 10: 95–109 (1976).

71 Ville de Goyet, C. de; Jeannée, E.: Epidemiological data on morbidity and mortality following the Guatemalan earthquake. Soc. Occ. Med. 4: 212 (1976).

72 Wallace, R.: Earthquake of August 19 1966, Varto area, eastern Turkey. Bull. seismol. Soc. Am. 38: 11 (1968); cited in Mitchell [51].

73 Western, K.A.: Report on PAHO activities after hurricane Liza, Baja, California Sur, Mexico (PAHO, Washington 1976).

74 Whittow, J.: Disasters (Allan Lane, London 1979).

75 Willis, M.F.: Case study of the 1974 Darwin cyclone disaster. Joint IHF/ IUA/UNDRO/WHO Seminar, Manila 1978.

76 Whittaker, R.; Fareed, D.; Green, P.; Barry, P.; Borge, A.: Fletes-Barrios earthquake disaster in Nicaragua – reflections on the initial management of massive casualties. J. Trauma 14: 37–43 (1974).

77 Winchester, P.: Disaster relief operations in Andhra Pradesh, southern India, following the cyclone in November 1977. Disasters 3: 173–178 (1979).

2. Communicable Disease and Disease Control after Natural Disasters

Introduction

Historically, epidemics of typhus, plague, dysentery, smallpox and other diseases have been a regular concomitant of war, famine and social upheavals. Perhaps for this reason, it is still widely believed that populations affected by natural disasters face a similar hazard from disease.

Paradoxically, observations after natural disasters suggest that major outbreaks of serious communicable diseases are uncommon. In part, this may reflect a lack of systematic observation of disease after disaster and in part the effectiveness of public health interventions during relief operations. Chiefly, however, it appears to reflect the comparative rarity of major population movements and other effects of disaster which would increase disease transmission.

However, it may also be concluded that there is a potential for the epidemic spread of disease after most major natural disasters, particularly in the developing countries, and that disease surveillance and other public health measures deemed necessary should be given a high priority in relief operations.

This chapter has been divided into three main parts: (1) a discussion of those effects of natural disasters which may influence the transmission of disease; (2) a review of the literature regarding disease experience after natural disasters, and (3) a brief description of the appropriate relief strategy for the control of communicable disease. The first part is based mainly on an account by *Western* [37].

Factors Affecting Disease Transmission after Natural Disasters

The transmission of communicable disease after natural disasters may be influenced by six main factors: (a) the diseases present in the population before a disaster and the endemic levels of disease; (b) ecological changes resulting from a disaster (e.g. the creation of new vector-breeding sites); (c) population movements; (d) damage to public utilities; (e) the disruption of disease control programmes, and (f) altered individual resistance to disease.

Preexisting Disease in the Population

Throughout history, warfare, famine and social upheavals have been closely associated with epidemics of louse-borne typhus and relapsing fever, plague, smallpox, cholera, shigella and other dysenteries, typhoid and paratyphoid fevers and tuberculosis. Until the turn of this century, there have probably been more deaths in warfare attributable to disease than to military activity; during famine in Europe until the mid-19th century and in the developing countries until the present day, the effects of starvation have usually been aggravated by or exceeded by the effects of disease.

Perhaps because of this type of association, it is still widely believed that the epidemic diseases of earlier times present a general threat to populations affected by natural disasters. Following many major natural disasters in both the industrialized and developing countries, rumours of epidemics (typically of well-known disease entities such as plague, typhoid, cholera and rabies) circulate amongst the survivors. Of more importance, great efforts have been directed by relief agencies at hastily organized immunization programmes, most often against typhoid fever and cholera.

Clearly, however, the risk of epidemic after a disaster is related to endemic levels of disease in the population: where a disease agent did not exist in a population before a disaster, there is generally no risk of an outbreak occurring. During this century, there have been enormous changes in the pattern of occurrence and the significance of diseases throughout the world – changes which have considerably altered the hazards of disease after natural disasters. In the industrialized countries, improved economic conditions, high levels of immunization against common diseases, improved water supplies and other public health interventions, as well as general access to effective curative services have eliminated many former scourges and dramatically reduced the importance of many others. In the developing countries, levels of communicable disease have remained high, and in general, are still the leading cause of morbidity and mortality. Even in these countries, however, ecological changes and public health activities have dramatically altered patterns of disease. Some diseases, such as smallpox, have been eradicated; some, such as louse-borne typhus and relapsing fever, have been reduced to relatively small areas in remote regions; and others, such as malaria, have been eradicated in some areas and partially controlled elsewhere.

At the same time, other diseases have increased in importance. Since 1961 cholera has spread widely in southeast Asia and to much of sub-Saharan Africa where it remains intermittently epidemic, whereas the Americas remain free of the disease. Shigella dysenteries have caused massive epidemics in Central America; in Guatemala for example, over 8,000 deaths occurred in 1969 – enough to make the disease a 'disaster' in its own right [14].

Such changes in the pattern of disease occurrence in different regions of the world lead to two main implications for disease control after disasters: (1) the probability of a disease outbreak after disaster is likely to be greater in the developing countries than in the industrialized regions; and (2) in most developing countries which are subject to natural disasters, the chief hazard from disease is not from the diseases previously associated with 'disasters'. The diseases now of most importance are those which are the common currency of poverty and low levels of public health activity throughout the developing world. These include the many etiological types of diarrhea and dysentery, measles, whooping cough and diphtheria, respiratory infections, meningococcal meningitis, intestinal parasites, scabies and other skin diseases, tuberculosis, and in many regions of the world, malaria.

Obviously, a potential for epidemics of diseases such as louse-borne typhus, relapsing fever and cholera would exist where these are endemic, e.g. these diseases were responsible for many deaths during the 1972/73 Ethiopian famine [20]. In many areas of the world, such diseases present little or no hazard following natural disasters.

Ecological Changes Resulting from Natural Disasters

Natural disasters may alter the potential for disease transmission by altering ecological conditions. In this context, the most important diseases are those transmitted by mosquito vectors and by water.

Vector-borne disease, and perhaps most importantly malaria, may increase as a result of a rise in the number of mosquito breeding sites and from the increased exposure of the population to the vector from loss of housing. In practise, the range of conditions which might occur after a disaster, and the wide variation in the breeding and biting habits of the many species of *Anopheles* mosquitoes which may transmit malaria are such as to make generalization about these effects impossible. For instance, *Western* [37] has pointed out that heavy rains occurring on the Caribbean coast of Central America might reduce the numbers of *A. aquasalis* which prefer brackish water as a breeding site, and increase the numbers of *A. albimanus* and *A. darlingi* which prefer fresh water, with unpredictable results on patterns of disease. A documented outbreak of malaria following a hurricane in Haiti in 1963 is discussed later in this chapter.

Culex mosquito species are in some areas the vectors of St. Louis and Japanese B encephalitis and bancroftian filariasis. *C. qinquefaciatus* breeds in pit latrines and other polluted water, breeding sites which might increase in camps and temporary settlements after disasters [12]; other *Culex* species might be increased by floods.

Increases in the mosquito population were noted after the hurricane ('Beulah') which struck Texas in 1967, and after the 1976 cyclone and storm-surge disaster in Andhra Pradesh in southern India [11, 25].

Reservoirs of plague are widely distributed in wild rodents, from which they may from time-to-time infect commensal rat populations in human communities. Man may be infected from flea bites or from contact with infected carcasses, conditions which might be increased by disasters: it is possible that the breakdown in living conditions which follows disasters in some urban areas might increase the hazard of pneumonic (man-to-man) plague transmission, but this hazard seems remote. After the earthquake in Agadir, Morocco in 1963, it was noted that large numbers of rats emerged from sewers. Cases of plague had been noted in the region some years before the earthquake [13].

The epidemic spread of louse-borne typhus depends upon the existence of a heavy infestation of a population with head or body lice, crowded living conditions and an endemic focus of disease. The distribution of louse-borne typhus in the world is shrinking and in most areas of the world these conditions are unlikely to be met after disaster. Similar considerations apply to the spread of louse-borne relapsing fever.

Many other diseases transmitted by arthropod vectors, including leishmaniasis, other rickettsial disease (e.g. murine and scrub typhus), and most anthropod-borne viral diseases are unlikely to present a hazard after natural disasters. Most of these diseases occur in remote and sparsely populated areas, or have little or no tendency to epidemic spread. They are chiefly a hazard to military rather than civilian populations [37].

The incidence of dog bites may increase after earthquakes, accompanied in many areas by an increased risk of rabies, as neglected strays come into close contact with persons living in temporary shelters. One such case, described later in this chapter, occurred following the 1976 Guatemala earthquake. Conjunctivitis, shigella dysentery, enterovirus infections and some parasitic diseases may be transmitted by domestic flies, which might be expected to increase in numbers after a disaster as a result of increased breeding in faeces and garbage.

Disease may also be transmitted by flood water. Leptospirosis is a disease of worldwide distribution which is spread by rodents, dogs, pigs, cattle and other wild animals. The disease is common in sewage workers and other occupations involving contact with infected water. Two outbreaks of leptospirosis associated with floods are described later in this chapter.

Other water-borne disease might also be spread by floods, although in practice the risk is probably reduced by the enormous dilution of contaminating sources by the volume of flood water. The risk of typhoid fever outbreaks from such contamination would seem to be small, as the typhoid bacterium does not multiply in water. Furthermore, people may be reluctant to drink from visibly contaminated water or from water imagined to be contaminated, and may seek safer sources of supply.

After floods in Zagreb, Yugoslavia in 1964, 660 swabs were taken from 220 randomly-selected dwellings 2–3 days after the flood: a further 120 swabs were taken from 40 sample sites in the dwellings of 10 typhoid and paratyphoid carriers living in the flooded area. *Salmonella meleagridis* was isolated from one sample; *S. typhi* and *S. paratyphi* were not isolated [6].

Population Movements

Population movements may influence the transmission of disease by increasing population density, thereby increasing the burden on the water supply and other services in the receiving area, and/or by introducing a susceptible population to a new disease or disease vector.

Population density is a critical factor in the transmission of disease from person-to-person, by vectors, or through the contamination of water and food. Serious outbreaks of disease are certain to occur only in areas where population density has increased without a commensurate increase in the provision of water supply, sanitation, immunization and other basic services. This has primarily been the experience of the many refugee movements which have occurred in Africa and Asia during the past decade, rather than after natural disasters [30].

The most important diseases to occur in temporary settlements and camps are diarrheal disease and dysentery, measles, whooping cough, malaria, tuberculosis, scabies and other skin infections. Children under the age of 5 years are most affected, often whith heavy mortality.

The lack of observations of outbreaks of this kind after natural disasters appears to reflect both the comparative rarity of major population displacements after disasters in the developing countries, and to some extent, the effectiveness of the public health measures which have been taken.

Some aspects of population movements after natural disasters are reviewed in chapter 3. After earthquakes, large intra-urban population movements may occur, as people who have lost their houses move to live with relatives and friends in undamaged areas, e.g. the movement of 200,000 people from Managua, Nicaragua following the 1972 earthquake [8]. People seeking shelter may also utilize schools and other public buildings. After some earthquakes, large 'squatter' settlements have grown up very rapidly, e.g. 50,000 improvised dwellings were erected within 24 h of the 1976 Guatemalan earthquake. People may also be moved into organized camps by the relief authorities. This occurred after the 1963 Agadir, Morocco earthquake where 15,000 people were moved into three camps [13]; after the 1967 floods at Varanasi, India where 3,000 people and 1,000 cattle were accommodated in a stadium [15]; after the 1972 earthquake in Nicaragua and the 1974 hurricane in Honduras where several small camps were erected [10]; and after the 1974 cyclone in Darwin, Australia where 6,000 people camped in and around a school [18]. The absence of serious outbreaks of disease in these instances was presumably related to the provision of basic services.

Population movements may also bring people into contact with a disease or a disease vector not prevalent in their home area. For example, a population may be moved from an area with no malaria to an area where it is endemic, as occurred during the movement of refugees across the Thai/Kampuchean border in 1979 [16].

Alternatively, displaced people might bring a disease or disease vector with them. This could be a problem in populations evacuated inland from a coastal area before a cyclone.

International relief workers who fail to protect themselves often fall victim to infectious hepatitis, malaria and other diseases. Relief workers or relief supplies might also conceivably introduce a disease into an area, or transport a disease vector to an area where it had been eradicated, e.g. a new strain of influenza, salmonella infection from relief foods, or a mosquito vector.

Damage to Public Utilities

Damage to water supply and sewage disposal systems has a clear potential for increasing levels of disease after many types of natural disaster. Failure of a pumped water system might cause a population to utilize other contaminated sources, or breaks in a water supply system might allow sewage contamination of the water with subsequent introduction of disease to a large population. That these effects have rarely been observed after natural disasters presumably reflects the adequacy of emergency repairs, hyperchlorination, increased pumping to maintain water pressure and other emergency measures taken by water authorities in both industrialized and developing countries [1, 4, 19, 26]. It also reflects the comparative rarity of piped water systems in rural and small urban areas of disaster-prone developing countries. Where the usual water source is a well, and sanitation by the use of pit latrines or fields, earthquakes would not be expected to result in water contamination, although there might be a risk of water contamination during floods. A survey of 18 remote sites following the 1976 Guatemalan earthquake found only one with a reported shortage of water [36].

The potential for disease spread through reticulated water systems, however, is amply illustrated by epidemics which have resulted from sewage contamination of water systems under non-disaster conditions, e.g. the 1963 outbreak of typhoid fever in Zermatt, Switzerland which caused 437 cases [7] and numerous outbreaks elsewhere [35]. Contamination of a piped water system was detected in 1971 after floods in Chester, Pennsylvania; however, there was no indication of a source of contamination within the flooded area and doubts were expressed about the quality of bacteriological monitoring [5]. 'Water pollution' was identified in Potenza after the 1980 earthquake in southern Italy [2]. The 1972 Managua, Nicaragua earthquake caused extensive damage to the water distribution system, reducing the number of connections from 38,000 before the earthquake to

17,200 afterwards. Although pumped water volume was rapidly restored and the quality of water sources was considered to be good, no bacteriological tests were conducted [19]. After the 1976 Guatemala earthquake, in which the main waterworks in the capital were extensively damaged, daily checks of bacteriological quality by the water authority were said to be within accepted norms; again, though doubts arose about the accuracy of the tests employed. Bacterial contamination was said to have been detected in emergency tanks supplied to temporary settlements [36].

Interruption of Public Health Services

In many developing countries, a range of potentially serious diseases are held in check by public health programmes, which, if interrupted by disaster, might lead to an outbreak of disease. Of most importance in this context are vector control programmes which might lead to a resurgence of malaria or other diseases, and routine immunization programmes against measles, whooping cough, poliomyelitis and diphtheria. The interruption of ambulatory tuberculosis programmes might also facilitate the spread of disease.

Altered Individual Resistance to Disease

Protein-energy malnutrition, which affects a variable proportion of children in the poorer populations of most developing countries, increases individual susceptibility to, and is aggravated by, many communicable diseases. In theory, this might increase the disease hazard after disaster in the developing countries. Observations by *Murray* et al. [24] in Somalian refugee camps in the Ethiopian Ogaden in 1975 suggest that refeeding malnourished individuals increased the incidence of several common infections, including malaria and tuberculosis.

Observations of Disease after Natural Disasters

Strikingly, records of the effects of natural disasters rarely report outbreaks of communicable disease.

This section is concerned with two qualitatively different types of disease reports, after natural disaster. The first is an account of those outbreaks of disease which have been reported after natural disasters. The second is a description of four published examples of organized disease surveillance after natural disasters, in which a systematic attempt has been made to estimate changes in levels of disease in a population.

Reported Outbreaks of Disease after Natural Disasters

Two outbreaks of leptospirosis have been reported, both related to floods. The first of these occurred in Lisbon, Portugal in 1967 although the number of cases was not reported. In previous floods in the city, no cases of the disease had been seen, and although the flood waters were said to be grossly contaminated during the 1967 flood, no other cases of water-borne diseases were recorded [31].

The second reported outbreak of leptospirosis occurred after floods in Greater Recife, Brazil, following floods in July 1975. Of 107 recorded cases, 105 were confirmed by seroagglutination or hemoculture. *Icterohaemorrhagiae* was the predominent serotype, found in 96 cases. Two previous outbreaks of leptospirosis occurred in Greater Recife in 1966 and 1970, although it is not clear whether these were also associated with floods [9].

To these two accounts may be added an outbreak of an unspecified fever after the 1978 cyclone in Sri Lanka [28], the aggravation of a preexisting typhoid fever problem in Mauritius after a hurricane, cases of food poisoning in Dominica and the Dominican Republic and the observation by physicians after disasters in industrialized countries of an apparent increase in minor respiratory infections, influenza and nonspecific diarrheas [37]. No other details are available on these outbreaks. After the 1977 cyclone and storm-surge disaster in Andhra Pradesh, southern India, 2,150 cases of gastroenteritis were recorded with 18 deaths: 6 cases of cholera were also confirmed bacteriologically. These diseases are endemic to the area and it is not clear if this represents an increased level of disease [11]. The only detailed study of a disease outbreak after a disaster is of an epidemic of malaria in Haiti following a hurricane, an account of which follows.

Malaria Epidemic in Haiti following a Hurricane [23].

On the night of October 3/4 1963, hurricane Flora crossed the southern peninsula of Haiti, directly affecting an area of approximately 2,200 km². Between 4,000 and 5,000 people were estimated to have been killed out of a population of 520,000 living in the area. Almost all houses in the area were destroyed, leaving 200,000 homeless. In addition to damage caused by the wind, further damage resulted from flooding caused by heavy rains, first on the night of the hurricane, and later on October 8 as the hurricane passed to the north of the island. The population of the area is predominantly rural with only about 10% living in small urban settlements.

Surveys conducted in 1960/61 of the area affected by the hurricane showed that malaria parasite rates were, in different localities, in the range 17–32%. Earlier surveys had shown that 88% of infections were due to *Plasmodium falciparum.* The principal vector was *A. albimanus,* mainly a coastal mosquito which spreads inland when conditions are suitable. The mosquito, although largely non-domestic and zoophilic does bite humans and will enter houses. Malaria transmission was considered to occur mainly in areas less than 500 m in altitude. The area affected by the hurricane is made up of two coastal plains separated by a discontinuous chain of highlands.

At the time of the hurricane, a malaria eradication programme was underway in Haiti. The programme began in March 1961, with the first DDT spraying of houses in January 1962: spraying was then repeated on a 6-monthly cycle. About 50% of the 4th spraying cycle was complete when the hurricane struck. In June 1962, 5 months after the beginning of the spraying operation, a malaria surveillance programme began. By October 1, 1963, 100 voluntary collaborator posts were in operation in the area affected by the hurricane. These posts were visited monthly by eight malaria service case-finders who also collected blood slides, mainly from localities along roads between collaborator posts.

The first sign of an unusual increase in malaria was a report by a post in mid-December 1963 of a sudden rise in the number of fever cases. The percentage of malaria-positive slides taken rose from 2% in September 1963 to 25.6% by the end of February 1964 (fig. 1). This increase apparently occurred simultaneously throughout the affected area. The percentage of positive slides then fell to 6.7% in May, followed by a second rise in July. At the height of the epidemic, approximately 10,000 slides were taken each month.

The highest positive slide rates were seen in children under 1 year (35.3%) although rates were also high in adults over 21 years of age (17.5%). The sexes were equally affected. Coastal areas showed higher rates than the interior and localities under 300 m altitude showed higher rates than higher altitudes. The percentage of cases with a high parasite density (more than 1,000 parasites mm^3 of blood) also rose, from 56% in October 1963 to 84% in June 1964. The outbreak was caused by *P. falciparum* which occurred in 98.6% of cases.

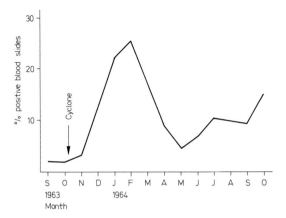

Fig. 1. Percent of malaria-positive blood slides by month in zone affected by the 1963 Haitian hurricane. Drawn from data in *Mason* et al. [23].

A first quick survey of housing losses, conducted at the end of October 1963 showed that approximately 68% of housing had been destroyed and the rest damaged to some degree. The 4th spraying cycle was therefore discontinued, as there was little housing left to spray. By December, about 80% of houses had been rebuilt or repaired and by the end of April 1964 reconstruction was virtually complete. Spraying was resumed on January 6, 1964.

It was estimated that about 75,000 cases of malaria occurred in the hurricane area between October 1963 and March 1964, based on an overall 25% positivity rate for fever cases with an estimated 50% of the population affected by fever during the course of the epidemic. Although mortality reporting in the area was poor, it was felt that little excess mortality resulted.

The epidemic was attributed to a combination of five factors: (1) as malaria transmission had not been interrupted by earlier spraying operations, there was a large reservoir of gametocyte carriers at the time of maximum mosquito activity after the hurricane; (2) there was a lack of shelter which resulted in a greater exposure of the population to the principal vector; (3) there was almost complete removal of insecticide from houses by the heavy rains; (4) there was an explosive increase in mosquito breeding due to heavy rainfall and flooding; (5) and there was increased population movement in search of food, construction materials, etc.

The failure of the spraying operation in early 1964 to prevent a second rise in the incidence of malaria was attributed to heavy rains during April, equal in amount to those during the hurricane, and to the probability that most malaria transmission occurred away from houses.

Disease Surveillance after Natural Disasters

The objective of disease surveillance after disaster is to identify disease outbreaks in order to investigate them and, if necessary, to instigate appropriate disease control measures.

The collection of information on disease is usually based upon the organization of a centralized system for monitoring the numbers of visits to hospitals and other medical facilities within the affected area. In the industrialized countries, reports may often be obtained by telephone and by utilizing existing channels for disease notification. In the developing countries, formidable difficulties may have to be overcome. In some instances, information may be obtained only with the aid of helicopters or surveillance teams willing to travel on foot. In addition to reports from medical facilities, it is also common practice to monitor the local press and media for reports of disease and to take into account other independent reports including rumors of epidemics. Where clinical facilities are inadequate in number or distribution to provide an adequate basis for reporting, sample surveys may be required to collect information.

The diseases considered for surveillance include those known to be endemic to the area in question, those which represent a serious health hazard and those which, if identified, are amenable to control. In the provincial areas of most developing countries, laboratory facilities are, even in normal times, inadequate to enable the accurate diagnosis of many diseases. Information is therefore usually collected in the form of symptoms or signs which suggest diseases of concern (e.g. fever and diarrhea, jaundice); in the case of clinically, easily-diagnosed conditions, presumptive diagnoses are made (e.g. measles). In some cases, information is also collected on trauma, malnutrition or other relevant conditions.

The interpretation of data collected in this way presents obvious difficulties. Changes in attendance at medical facilities are not necessarily representative of changes in the levels of disease in the general population. In most countries, comparable baseline data are lacking; even where available, patterns of attendance may be distorted by damage to existing facilities and by the introduction of new relief reporting stations. Nevertheless, such reports may indicate the presence of serious disease, such as typhoid fever, or show sufficiently clear trends to warrant further local investigation.

The four published accounts of disease surveillance after natural disasters are described below.

The East Bengal Cyclone and Storm-Surge, November 12–13, 1970.
This cyclone and storm-surge affected a large area of coastal East Bengal, and caused a mortality of 16.5% representing a minimum of 224,000 deaths. After the cyclone, two surveys were conducted by *Sommer and Mosely* [33]. The first survey, conducted 2–3 weeks after the cyclone served to estimate immediate relief needs. The second survey, conducted after a delay of 2 months, was designed to serve as a basis for long-term planning for relief and recovery. An area which had not been affected by the cyclone was also surveyed as a control [see also chap. 1, p. 36].

On the first rapid survey, all injured and ill at each of 18 sample sites were examined; rivers, ponds and open wells, the usual sources of drinking water, were also tested for saline content by electrical conductivity. The second survey was concentrated in the most severely affected area. Two villages were studied in each of the 72 unions (the smallest administrative division). 20 nonadjacent families were interviewed in each sample village.

The results of the first survey showed that in all areas except one, where the water was almost undrinkable (0.25–0.5% saline) the salt content was always found to be less than 0.1%. In most areas the salinity of surface water was comparable to water from shallow artesian wells. No evidence was found on this survey of any excess of smallpox (at that time an endemic disease in Bengal), cholera, other diarrheal diseases or respiratory tract infections.

On the second survey, post-cyclone mortality and morbidity were found to be comparable with norms in Bengal. Mortality during the first 3-month period after the disaster ranged from 0.2 to 0.6% in different areas, compared with 0.5% in the control area. Age-specific post-cyclone mortality for the cyclone and control areas were found to be similar, except for a higher mortality amongst middle-aged residents of the control area. This was probably attributable to the elimination of sickly middle-aged individuals from the population during the cyclone [see also chap. 1, p. 38]. Post-cyclone morbidity was 'confined primarily to the usual diarrheal and respiratory tract diseases'.

The 1972 Earthquake in Managua, Nicaragua [8]

On December 23, 1972, an earthquake severely damaged Managua, the capital of Nicaragua, causing approximately 4,000 deaths and 20,000 injuries in a population of approximately 400,000. Earthquake damage was essentially confined to the urban area of the capital.

After the earthquake, all hospitals and clinics in the city were required to report daily suspected or diagnosed cases of typhoid fever, diarrheal disease, deaths (and their cause) and other significant or unusual disease occurrences. According to *Coultrip* [8] there were no cases of typhoid fever or abnormal levels of gastroenteritis.

The 1976 Earthquake in Guatemala [29, 34].

The 1976 earthquake in Guatemala affected one-third of the area of the country resulting in approximately 23,000 deaths and 77,000 injuries. An emergency disease surveillance programme was initiated on the second day after the earthquake in the most heavily damaged area and continued until the 19th post-earthquake day. A permanent surveillance system was then established which continued for a further year. During the emergency phase, information collection was limited to only two of the four earthquake-affected departments because the relief authorities wished to concentrate efforts on the areas of greatest population and destruction.

In Guatemala City, the capital, information was collected daily from the registration forms of patients attending 7 main medical facilities. Information was also collected retrospectively for the day before and the day after the earthquake. In the rural areas, information was collected by community health workers and nursing aids. In two rural areas, the records of 12 public health centers and hospitals were also surveyed during the period 15–19 days after the earthquake.

Categories of diseases reported included trauma, upper respiratory tract infections, fever without rash or cough and 'others'. In addition, diagnoses of typhoid fever, measles, pertussis, dog bite, rabies, meningitis, tetanus, poliomyelitis, dysentery and enteritis, pneumonia and malnutrition were also extracted from records of medical consultations. Bacteriological laboratories continued to function in Guatemala City which were used to follow-up reports of typhoid fever and shigellosis in the city. In addition, some 30 rumours of disease outbreaks, including measles, typhoid fever, anthrax, rabies, hepatitis, influenza and dysentery were investigated.

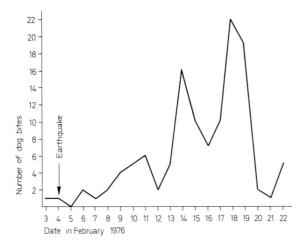

Fig. 2. Daily hospital attendances for dog bites in Guatemala City after the 1976 earthquake. Data read from published graph in *Spencer* et al. [34].

No increase in the absolute number or proportion of attendances for diarrhea, or fever without rash or cough was seen. The proportion of attendances for upper respiratory tract infection increased, but as this pattern was common for February and March and a similar pattern was observed in non-earthquake-affected areas, it was not considered to be a result of the earthquake. A small increase in the number of cases of malnutrition was observed between weeks 14 and 31 post-earthquake. It was felt that this probably represented only a larger number of people coming to free food distribution points rather than an increase in the prevalence of malnutrition [see chap. 4, p. 91].

The only clear increase in any diagnostic category was of dog bites, which occurred in the second post-earthquake week in all areas of Guatemala City (see fig. 2). Although no cases of rabies were reported, the Ministry of Health began a programme for the elimination of stray dogs. Increased numbers of dog bites in the second week after earthquakes have also been observed following other earthquakes in Latin America [34][1].

---

[1] An increased incidence of snake bite has been reported from Malaysia during floods, as both snakes and the human population converged on limited areas of high ground [22].

The Earthquake of November 1980 in Southern Italy [17]

On November 23, 1980 an earthquake caused extensive damage in the regions of Campania and Basilicata in southern Italy. There were 2,459 recorded deaths and 7,173 recorded injuries. Naples was heavily damaged and in the city alone, 100,000 people were left homeless.

After the earthquake, a disease surveillance system was established. This was based on records of admissions (not including outpatient consultations) of earthquake 'survivors' at 52 hospitals in the area, a 'survivor' being defined as an individual who resided in one of the 315 communities within a government-defined emergency area. Information was collected daily from the 14th day after the earthquake until the 91st day, and weekly thereafter until the 27th post-earthquake week. For the first 14 post-earthquake days, data were collected retrospectively from hospital records. 16 categories of admissions were recorded, including viral hepatitis, typhoid fever, meningitis, measles, whooping cough, diarrhea with and without fever, and cough with fever.[2] This information was stratified into two age groups, 0–15 years and 16 years and over. In addition, information on 20 specific communicable diseases was collected every 10 days from 4 provincial medical officers in the earthquake area. All information collected was computer processed. Where a cluster of disease was suspected, diagnosis was checked by telephone with the admitting hospital and a local epidemiologist was sent to investigate. Disease notifications from provincial medical officers were compared with records of the same disease categories for the equivalent 10-day period from each of the preceding 3 years.

Surveillance of hospital admissions showed small absolute numbers of admissions (2–3 admissions/week) and a static trend for admissions for

---

[2] Information was also collected for admissions for psychological disturbances, hypothermia and frostbite, trauma (including injuries incurred after the earthquake), general surgery, general medicine, obstetrics and gynecology and for social reasons. Admissions for psychological disorders fell sharply from approximately 40 in the first post-earthquake week (week 1) to 10 by week 5, and fell slowly thereafter to 5 admissions/week by week 23. Hypothermia and frostbite showed a less clear trend: 8 cases had been admitted by week 6, a further 11 cases in weeks 7–10, and 3 cases more in weeks 11–27. Admissions for trauma fell sharply from approximately 1,000 in week 1 to 300 in week 3 and remained roughly constant until week 27. General surgical and obstetric/gynecological admissions rose from 400 and 200 admissions respectively in week 1 to approximately constant levels of 600 and 400 admissions/week in week 7 and remained roughly constant until week 27. Admissions for social reasons totalled approximately 25 by week 11: approximately 70 more admissions were made by week 15. There were no further admissions until week 25 when 110 cases were admitted.

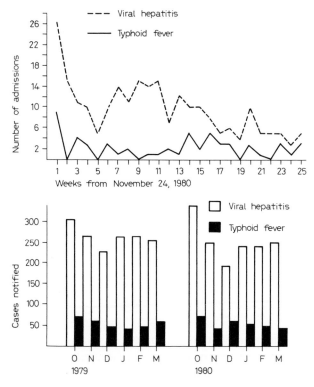

Fig. 3. Graph of weekly hospital admissions for viral hepatitis and typhoid fever after the 1980 earthquake in southern Italy. Histogram of monthly notifications of viral hepatitis and typhoid fever for the 2 months before, and the 4 months after the earthquake, and for the same period in 1979. Data read from published graph in *Greco* et al. [17].

measles, meningococcal meningitis and whooping cough. Admissions for cough with fever also showed a static trend.

The difficulty of interpreting trends in hospital admissions is illustrated by figures 3 and 4. Figure 3 shows hospital admissions by week for viral hepatitis and typhoid fever, contrasted with monthly figures for notifications for the same diseases during the earthquake period and for the same period in the preceding year: figure 4 shows weekly admissions for diarrhea with and without fever. From figure 3 it can be seen that the number of cases notified is substantially greater than the number admitted

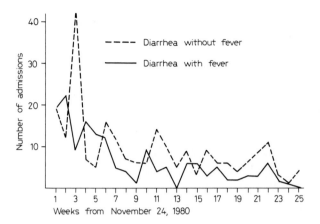

Fig. 4. Weekly admissions for diarrhea with and without fever after the 1980 earthquake in southern Italy. Data read from published graph in *Greco* et al. [17].

for each diagnosis. The negative trends apparent in admissions for diarrheal disease might reflect a real change in disease incidence or merely changes in patterns of hospital attendance or admission.

A further statistical analysis of the original surveillance data by *Alexander* [3] showed that: (i) between July 1978 and October 1980 (pre-earthquake) there was wide variation between months in notifications of viral hepatitis, typhoid and paratyphoid fevers, and meningococcal meningitis, making it difficult to estimate mean values with precision: this difficulty was aggravated by a significant decline in the reported incidence of typhoid fever during the same period. Rates of viral hepatitis, paratyphoid fever and meningococcal meningitis had remained stable; (ii) with these reservations in mind, comparison of the data for the 28 pre-earthquake months with that from the 7 post-earthquake months showed that the notifications of viral hepatitis and typhoid fever were significantly lower after the disaster. There was no significant difference in the incidence rates of meningitis or paratyphoid fever.

During the 27 weeks of surveillance, there were 32 suspected epidemics. Of these only two were confirmed: one consisted of 39 cases of gastroenteritis in a group of firemen, and the other of 6 cases of viral hepatitis in the province of Potenza, on the edge of the earthquake zone.

Disease Control after Natural Disasters

After many recent natural disasters in both the industrialized and developing countries, local and international relief agencies have been preoccupied with the risk of epidemics. Major concerns have usually been with the organization of immunization programmes, usually against typhoid fever and cholera, and with the disposal of corpses and animal carcasses which are seen as a probable focus for disease outbreaks [2, 21, 27, 34].

To a large extent, these concerns arise from the inexperience of relief personnel, although in some cases the relief authorities may feel under political pressure from the population to be seen to be active in disease control. Donated vaccines are often available in large quantities and immunization programmes provide a convenient, easily organized, 'high visibility' activity. *Gurd* [18] for example, has defended the decision to conduct immunization against typhoid and tetanus after the 1974 cyclone in Darwin, Australia, as a means of both protecting the population against a disease risk and of raising public morale.

The technical objections to this approach to disease control are obvious. The risk of typhoid fever or cholera may be very small in comparison to other diseases; the vaccines are only partly effective; it is rarely possible to obtain more than partial population coverage with a single dose of vaccine in a hastily-organized programme; the costs are considerable; personnel are diverted from more useful activities; and there may be a significant rate of vaccine reactions. Corpses and animal carcasses, unless contaminating water supplies, are an unlikely focus for epidemic disease. At worst, they present a risk to body handlers, and then only if minimal hygienic precautions are not taken. There are of course other reasons for the rapid disposal of corpses and carcasses, such as the direct offence and the hazard from flies and rodents, particularly in tropical climates. However, the precipitate disposal of human remains by mass cremation or burial and the use of lime as a disinfectant may be hygienically unnecessary and may hinder the identification of bodies [32].

During the past decade, experience has shown that there is a more practical and effective approach to disease control after natural disasters. This involves two lines of activity: The first is reducing the disease hazard by appropriate public health interventions, emphasizing primarily those areas which present the greatest risks. This may include the emergency repair of water supplies to urban areas, the provision of water supplies, emergency sanitation systems and immunization programmes, particularly against measles and whooping cough in camps and temporary settlements, and vector control operations. The second is establishing a surveillance system so that outbreaks of disease which do occur can be promptly identified and controlled. Detailed operational manuals describing this approach are now available [12, 37].

References

1   Adrian, G.W.; Goldman, A.; Forthal, A.A.: Water quality after a disaster. J. Am. Wat. Wks Ass. *63:* 481–485 (1972).

2   Alexander, D.: The earthquake of 23 November 1980 in Campania and Basilicata, Southern Italy (International Disaster Institute, London 1981).

3   Alexander, D.: Epidemiological surveillance of diseases following the earthquake of 23rd November 1980, in Southern Italy: discussion. Disasters *6:* 149–153 (1982).

4   Alter, A.J.: Environmental health experiences in disaster. Am. J. publ. Hlth *60:* 475–480 (1970).

5   Appleyard, V.A.; Hetzer, H.W.: Flooding in Chester, Pa. J. Am. Wat. Wks Ass. *64:* 480–481 (1973).

6   Bencic, Z.: Disinfection of dwellings after flooding (English abstract). Lijecn. Vjesn. *88:* 939–940 (1966).

7   Bernard, R.P.: The Zermatt typhoid outbreak in 1963. J. Hyg., Camb. *63:* 537–561 (1965).

8   Coultrip, R.L.: Medical aspects of US disaster relief operations in Nicaragua. Milit. Med. *139:* 879–883 (1974).

9   Continho de Oliveira, V.J.; Baracho da Rocha, J.M.; da Silva, G.B.; Cabral, C.L.N.: Considerations on the new epidemic outbreak of human leptospirosis in Greater Recife, Brazil in 1975. Disasters *5:* 46–48 (1981).

10 Cuny, F.C.: Refugee camps and camp planning: the state of the art. Disasters *1:* 125–143 (1977).

11 Dharmaraju, P.: Emergency health and medical care in cyclone and tidal wave affected areas of Andhra Pradesh. Joint IHF/IUA UNDRO/WHO Seminar, Manila 1978.

12 Emergency vector control after natural disaster. Scient. publ. No. 419 (Pan American Health Organization, Washington 1982).

13 Fernand, G.; Sentici, M.: Considerations sur les aspects sanitaires du seisme d'Agadir. Maroc. méd. *40:* 121–125 (1961).

14 Gangarosa, E.J.; Perera, D.R.; Mata, L.J.; Mendizabal-Morris, C.; Guzman, G.; Reller, L.B.: Epidemic shiga bacillus dysentery in Central America. II. Epidemiologic studies in 1969. J. infect. Dis. *122:* 181–190 (1970).

15 Gaur, S.D.; Marwash, S.M.: Public health aspects of floods with illustrations from 1967 Varanasi floods. Indian J. publ. Hlth *12:* 93–94 (1968).

16 Glass, R.I.; Cates, W.; Nieburg, P.; Davis, C.; Russbach, R.; Nothdurft, H.; Peel, S.; Turnbull, R.: Rapid assessment of health status and preventive medicine needs of newly arrived Kampuchean refugees, Sa Kaeo, Thailand. Lancet *i:* 868–872 (1980).

17 Greco, D.; Faustini, A.; Forastiere, F.; Galanti, M.R.; Magliola, M.E.; Moro, M.L.; Piergentili, P.; Rosmini, F.; Stazi, M.A.; Luzi, S.; Fantozzi, L.; Capocaccia, R.; Conti, S.; Zampieri, A.: Epidemiological surveillance of diseases following the earthquake of 23rd November 1980 in Southern Italy. Disasters 5: 398–406 (1981).

18 Gurd, C.H.: Public health aspects of natural disasters (unpubl. 1978).

19 Hazen, R.: Managua earthquake: some lessons in design and management. J. Am. Wat. Wks Ass. 66: 324–326 (1975).

20 Holt, J.; Seaman, J.: The scope of the drought, in Hussein, Rehab: drought and famine in Ethiopia. (International African Institute, London 1976).

21 Janik, F.; Hinze, E.: Hygienic measures and experiences in the flood catastrophe in Hamburg in 1962 (English abstract). Münch. med. Wschr. 104: 1987–1991 (1962).

22 Mackay, H.: Personal communication.

23 Mason, J.; Cavalie, P.: Malaria epidemic in Haiti following a hurricane. Am. J. trop. Med. Hyg. 14: 533–539 (1965).

24 Murray, M.J.; Murray, A.B.; Murray, M.B.; Murray, C.J.: Somali food shelters in the Ogaden famine and their impact on health. Lancet ii: 1283–1285 (1976).

25 Peavy, J.E.: Hurricane Beulah. Am. J. publ. Hlth 60: 481–484 (1970).

26 Phillips, R.V.: Los Angeles Earthquake of February 9, 1971. J. Am. Wat. Wks Ass. 64: 477–480 (1973).

27 Queen, C.R.; Stewart, R.S.: Physicians evaluate medical aspects, effectiveness of plans in Beulah. Tex. med. J. 63: 124–130 (1967).

28 Resstler, E.: Personal communication.

29 Romero, A.B.; Cobar, R.; Western, K.A.; Lopez, S.M.: Some epidemiological features of disasters in Guatemala. Disasters 2: 39–46 (1978).

30 Simmonds, S.P.; Gabaudan, M.: Refugee camp health care: selected annotated references. Ross Institute of Tropical Hygiene publ. No. 14 (London School of Hygiene and Tropical Medicine, London 1982).

31 Simoes, J.; Azevedeo, J.F.; Palmeiro, J.M.: Some aspects of the Weil's disease epidemiology based on a recent epidemic after a flood in Lisbon (1967) (English abstract). Anais Esc. nac. Saude publ. Med. trop 3: 19–32 (1969).

32 Skordic, S.: Comment on organization of hygienic measures applied in units of the Yugoslav army after the earthquake in Skoplje (English abstract). Vojno-sanit. Pregl. 21: 496–498 (1964).

33 Sommer, A.; Mosely, W.H.: East Bengal cyclone of November 1970 – epidemiological approach to disaster assessment. Lancet ii: 1029–1036 (1972).

34 Spencer, H.C.; Campbell, C.C.; Romero, A.; Zeissig, O.; Feldman, R.A.; Boostrom, E.R.; Croft Long, E.: Disease surveillance and decision-making after the 1976 Guatemala earthquake. Lancet i: 181–184 (1977).

35 Taylor, A.; Craun, G.F.; Faich, G.A.; McCabe, L.J.; Gangarosa, E.J.: Outbreaks of water-borne diseases in the United States, 1961–1970. J. infect. Dis. 132: 329–331 (1975).

36 Ville de Goyet, C., de; del Cid, E.; Romero, A.; Jeannee, E.; Lechat, M.: Earthquake in Guatemala – epidemiologic evaluation of the relief effort. Bull. Pan Am. Hlth Org. 10: 95–109 (1976).

37 Western, K.A.: Epidemiologic surveillance after natural disaster. Scient. publ. No. 420 (Pan American Health Organization, Washington 1982).

3. Environmental Exposure
after Natural Disaster

Introduction

Emergency shelter, clothing and blankets are widely regarded as life-saving relief items without which disaster victims run a high risk of death from environmental exposure. The objects of this chapter are to examine this belief and to lay down a framework within which the risk of environmental exposure can be assessed. (This discussion is limited to the topic of environmental exposure. The problem of the provision of shelter clearly raises much more complex issues. See for example *Davis* [10].)

Such a framework will have to be a theoretical one. There are no reliable reports in the literature of death from environmental exposure after any recent disaster on land. (There are rare reports of large numbers of deaths from exposure after some pre-war disasters, e.g. the Erzincan, Turkey earthquake of 1939 [2].) From this, it could be inferred that no exposure problem exists; but people dying of exposure after disaster are unlikely to do so in places where clinical facilities are sufficiently adequate to allow reliable certification of causes of death, and it cannot be assumed that no deaths from exposure have occurred.

The argument advanced in this chapter is that while theoretical considerations indicate that environmental exposure is a likely corollary of disasters, observations of the ability of survivors to protect themselves against the environment suggest that deaths from exposure after disaster are probably rare. On theoretical grounds, the major impact of exposure is an increased food requirement of the affected populations, and possibly an increased prevalence of protein-energy malnutrition (PEM). Paradoxically, this effect may be more important after disasters in warm countries than in temperate or cold regions.

Due to the lack of published observations directly relevant to environmental exposure after disasters, there are two approaches to this topic: (1) examination of the physiological effects of specific environmental conditions on individuals, and (2) examination of the known environmental conditions to which people are exposed after natural disasters.

A summary of the theoretical aspects of this topic, based on references [11, 17–19], is presented below.

The Physiology of Environmental Exposure

Humans, like all other mammals are homeotherms. That is, they regulate body temperature within a narrow range by balancing the heat produced by the metabolism of food with the heat lost or gained from the environment. The average western man, for example, eats about 3,000 kcal/day, of which about 95% is converted to heat. This is equivalent to heat production of approximately 2 kcal/h/kg of body weight, and if no heat were lost from the body, the body temperature would rise by about 2 °C/h.

The biological advantage of homeothermy is increased freedom from the environment. In conditions of environmental extremes, however, food requirements must be increased to keep the body warm, unless heat loss can be prevented. Heat may be lost from the body to the environment by four routes: radiation, conduction, convection and evaporation. Heat may be gained from the environment by radiation, conduction and convection. There is considerable variation regarding the importance of each of these routes under different environmental conditions.

Radiation
Like all other forms of radiation (e.g. light, radio or X-ray), radiant heat is an electromagnetic wave transmitted at the speed of light from a source to a receiver. All objects radiate heat towards cooler ones, regardless of the temperature of the air between them. The temperature of the surface of the human body varies widely, but may be approximated to 33 °C; only if the temperature of the surrounding environment is below this will heat be lost from the body by radiation.

Where there are 'hot-spots' in the environment, heat may be simultaneously gained and lost from the body by radiation. Examples of this are sitting by a camp fire on a cold night and direct exposure to the sun.

The rate of heat loss or gain by radiation for each unit area of body surface (the heat flux) over the range of environmental temperatures relevant to the discussion here, is approximately linearly proportional to the temperature difference between the body surface and the environment.

In practice, the amount of heat exchanged with the environment and the body by radiation depends not only upon the temperature gradient, but also upon the amount of skin exposed an the nature of the skin covering. Clothing lowers the surface temperature of the area it covers, which restricts losses; it also reflects incident radiation. For example, light-coloured clothing may reflect as much as 70% of the incident radiation, and being in the shade totally removes any derived radiative effect of the sun. Nevertheless, as anyone who has been exposed to a tropical sun can testify, heat loads from radiation can be immense: *Blum* [4], for example, has estimated that the average order of impact of sunlight on a nude man, assuming 43% reflection from blond skin, is about 240 kcal/h.

Heat losses by radiation are also quite variable, but, at lower temperatures, may account for 60–65% of all heat lost from the body [18].

Conduction

Conduction is the direct transfer of heat from one object to another with which it is in contact. The rate of heat loss by conduction is directly proportional to the temperature gradient between the two objects and their ability to conduct heat. Many household items are selected for their lack of conductivity (e.g. wood, clothing) and our lives are only made tolerable by the fact that the medium which surrounds us, air, has an extremely low conductivity. That is why, for example, room air at a temperature of 18 °C feels comfortably warm, while water, at the same temperature, feels cold.

Under ordinary conditions, conductive heat loss to the environment is small, but it is easy to imagine situations after disasters where this route of heat loss could become very important. For example, lying on a stone floor, or immersion in water below body temperature may enormously increase heat losses by conduction. An unclothed man of average build immersed in water at 5 °C will become helpless from hypothermia in 20–30 min; at 15 °C he would survive for 1.5–2 h.

The limit of voluntary tolerance of individuals to immersion (determined by the onset of nausea, malaise, cramps and cardiac dysrythmias) is related to skin and core temperature, and to the maximum production of heat by the body. *Boutelier* et al. [5] have shown that thin, nude subjects have a tolerance time of only 2 h in water at 26 °C. Death from hypothermia occurs when rectal temperature falls to approximately 25 °C.

Although conduction is not normally an important route of heat loss, it is of great importance in heat exchange within the body. Heat is lost from the surface of the body, and the rate of transmission of heat from the body core depends upon the conductivity of body tissues. Animal tissues are fairly good insulators (the thermal conductivity constant of human tissues is approximately 0.0005 cal/s/cm²/cm/°C, compared with, for example, glass with a constant of 0.0025 cal/s/cm²/cm/°C, or soft wood at 0.00009 cal/s/cm²/cm/°C).

Changes in blood flow modify the conductivity of tissues. A tenfold range in conductivity may be achieved by physiological variations in blood flow by vasodilation and vasoconstriction. These homeostatic mechanisms alter the temperature gradient that exists between the body core and the skin surface. Vasoconstriction increases the temperature gradient so that a lower skin temperature is maintained at any metabolic rate, and heat loss to the environment is reduced. Vasodilation has the opposite effect.

Clothing reduces heat loss to the environment by the same method. Normal western clothing has an insulation value of approximately 1 clo (the 'clo' is a unit of insulation defined as the amount of insulation which will allow the passage of 1 kcal/m²/h with a temperature gradient of 0.18 °C between the two sides) so that the surface temperature of clothing is lower than that of the skin; heat loss is correspondingly reduced.

Convection

Conductive heat loss, as mentioned, involves the flow of heat from the body to the surface with which it is in contact; convective heat loss involves the movement away from the body surface of that which has been warmed, i.e. the air or water with which the body is in contact.

The potential importance of convection to body heat loss is evident to anyone who has sat in a draft or in the wind. The rate of heat loss by this route has been shown to vary linearly with the difference between skin and air temperature, and with the square root of the wind speed.

This relationship enables the cooling effects of the wind to be quantified by expressing the effects of air speed on convective losses in terms of the changes in environmental temperature which would have the same impact. For example, a change in wind velocity from 0.9 m/s (3.2 km/h) to 4.5 m/s (16 km/h) has roughly the same effect on convective heat loss at 20 °C as a 4 °C fall in temperature. At lower temperatures, the effect is

Table I. Predicted lowest ambient temperature for prolonged thermal comfort

Bodily activity	Wind, sky, altitude	Predicted lowest ambient temperature for prolonged thermal comfort, °C		
		nude (0 clo)	business suit (1 clo)	arctic suit (4 clo)
Sitting quietly	no wind, shade, sea level	28	21	1
Sitting quietly	5 mph, shade, sea level	31	24	4
Sitting quietly	25 mph, shade, sea level	32	26	6
Sitting quietly	5 mph, sunshine, sea level	24	18	−2
Sitting quietly	5 mph, sunshine, 20,000 ft	19	12	−8
Walking 3.5 mph	5 mph, shade, sea level	25	12	−29

Modified from table given in *Newburgh* [19].

greater for a given wind speed. At 0 °C the same change in wind speed is equivalent to a 14 °C fall in temperature. Although these calculations are only approximations, neglecting the effects of wind speed and environmental temperatures on losses by other routes and assuming that skin temperature remains at a constant 31 °C, they do allow an understanding of the very great importance of the 'wind-chill factor' at even modest wind speeds. Table I shows the level of clothing insulation required for prolonged physical comfort under different environmental conditions. For example, for a person wearing 1 'clo', typical of many developing countries, in conditions of no wind and at rest, this is only possible at temperatures of 21 °C or more.

Evaporation
Water absorbs energy as it passes from the liquid to the gaseous state, termed the 'latent heat of evaporation'. The value for water is approximately 0.58 kcal/g at normal skin temperature. Water is evaporated from the body by three main routes: loss through expired air; passive diffusion through the skin, and active secretion onto the skin via the sweat glands.

The rate of the evaporative heat loss from the body depends upon the rate of water loss. The rate of removal of water by the ambient air depends upon the difference in the vapour pressure at the skin/air interface and that of the ambient air, and the velocity of wind flow. As with convection, evaporative losses vary with the square root of wind speed.

At environmental temperatures below skin temperature, losses of body heat by evaporation are small and remain essentially constant regardless of temperature and wind speed. In an adult this 'insensible water loss' amounts to approximately 30 g/h, equivalent to a heat loss of approximately 400 kcal/day. But as environmental temperatures rise above skin temperature, and heat cannot be lost from the body by other routes, evaporative losses through sweating become progressively more important.

Rates of sweating vary enormously under different environmental conditions. Experimentally, rates as high as 4 litres/h have been recorded: under more realistic conditions, e.g. men marching in direct sunlight at 40 °C, rates may be as high as 1 litre/h. Even sitting in the shade at the same temperature may cause sweating losses of 0.5 litre/h.

The body can adjust to only a small degree of dehydration, and losses of both water and salt must be replaced. The concentration of sodium chloride in the sweat of acclimatized subjects is about 1–1.5 g/litre.

The Concept of Thermoneutrality

The discussion so far has indicated that although heat must be lost from the body, an individual can, within limits, control the rate of heat loss by the physiological control of blood flow through the skin and by the control of sweating. By the control of heat loss, a range of environmental conditions is created within which heat production is in equilibrium with heat loss. This range of temperatures is called the thermoneutral zone (often defined as 'the range of ambient temperature within which metabolic rate is at a minimum, and within which temperature regulation is achieved by non-evaporative physical processes alone'; fig. 1).

If environmental temperature falls below the thermoneutral zone, the control of heat loss is no longer sufficient to maintain body temperature. Either the metabolic rate must rise or the body temperature must fall. The temperature at which a rise in metabolic rate is evident, is called the 'lower critical temperature (LCT)' (point B; fig. 1). Similarly, if the environmental

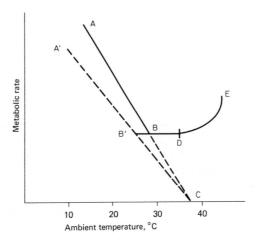

Fig. 1. Diagram to show the concept of thermoneutrality. Over the temperature range B/B′–D, heat production remains constant and minimal (thermoneutral zone). Below B/B′ and above D (UCT) heat production rises. The length of the zone of thermoneutrality (BD or B′D) is greater when the body insulation is greater: below B/B′ insulation can no longer conserve heat. Metabolism increases at a rate proportional to the gradient between core body temperature and ambient temperature. Line AB extrapolates to the core temperature (C) at zero metabolism; the greater the insulation, the flatter the slope (A′B′). Figure reproduced from *Maclean and Emslie-Smith* [18].

temperature rises, an 'upper critical temperature (UCT)' is reached, above which increased metabolic activity is required to regulate body temperature through sweating. Below the LCT, metabolic activity rises (through active work, sweating, and a process known as 'non-shivering thermogenesis') roughly linearly with falling temperatures; above the UCT, the relationship is non-linear.

Within the zone of thermoneutrality, therefore, a minimum of energy is expended on maintaining a constant body temperature, but above and below the critical temperatures, body temperature can only be maintained at the cost of extra energy consumption. At some point below the LCT, metabolic activity cannot expand sufficiently, and body temperature falls. Figure 2 shows the relationship between metabolic heat production, heat loss and deep-body temperature.

The values of the critical temperatures determined experimentally are not as precisely defined as figure 1 might indicate. Experiments in man tend to produce curvilinear relationships at the points of transition, rather

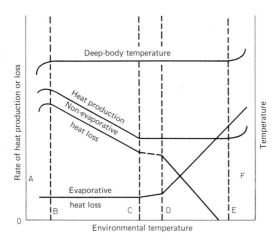

Fig. 2. Schematic representation between heat production, evaporative and non-evaporative heat loss and deep-body temperature in a homeothermic animal. A = Zone of hypothermia; B = temperature of peak metabolism and incipient hypothermia; C = critical temperature (LCT in fig. 1); D = temperature of marked rise in evaporative heat loss; E = temperature of incipient hyperthermal rise (UCT in fig. 1); F = zone of hyperthermia; CD-zone of least thermo-regulatory effort; CE-zone of minimal metabolism (thermoneutral zone in fig. 1). From *Mount* [17].

than the sharp inflections shown. Also, the actual values of the critical temperatures are not fixed, but vary according to the physique, age, body composition and insulation of the individual concerned. The slope of line AB in figure 1 is a measure of the level of insulation, i.e. as point A moves towards point A', the LCT, indicated by point B', falls.

Moreover, it is fictitious to imagine a person with a constant metabolic rate. Metabolic rate varies according to activity and food intake. It is minimal in a person who is fasting and resting, higher in a person who is not fasting and resting, and still higher in a non-fasting person taking exercise. As figure 1 makes clear, as metabolic rate falls, the LCT rises.

Given such limitations, the LCT for an adult male of typical European physique in the basal state (resting, fasting for 12–14 h) would be about 26–28 °C; light indoor clothing would lower this to about 24 °C, while light clothing and consumption of food at the average western level would lower it again to about 18 °C, or approximately room temperature. More realistically, in the context of disasters, which affect chiefly poor people in developing countries, where food intakes may be 60% of those in more affluent regions, values of the LCT would be increased to about 30 °C for a basal subject and 20 °C for a clothed one.

Can the Physiological and Nutritional Consequences of Environmental Exposure Be Predicted?

From the preceding section, it may seem that theoretically satisfying general relationships between body heat loss and the environment could be advanced, but unfortunately this cannot yet be done. Several conceptual and experimental problems arise, chiefly in the definition of the state of the individual.

Three main problems arise. First is the difficulty of predicting the vapour pressure of water at the skin surface except when high sweat rates leave the skin wetted. Second is the problem of determining the actual skin temperature, as the temperatures of different parts of the body vary. Finally, there is the problem of defining body surface area. The effective body surface for each route of heat loss is different, each differing from true anatomical surface area. For example, the radiating surface of an adult man may be only 70–80% of the anatomical surface (because of the areas of the body, such as the inner aspects of the thighs, which exchange radiation losses). The effective convective surface area is estimated at 80% of anatomical surface in the upright subject. In the upright position, the only important route of conduction loss is through the soles of the feet; in a subject sleeping on the ground, the area of contact is much larger, although even then it varies with the sleeping posture.

However, in spite of these difficulties, it must be stressed that there is sufficient information to define, within useful limits, the extent of the problems likely to be faced by survivors of disaster under different environmental conditions, even if it is not possible to assign precise quantities to the metabolic effects in any specific case. For example, the importance of air movement in heat loss is not just a question of gales, but even of slight air currents. Experiments in England have shown that in April, winds were severe enough to double the metabolic rate in one lightly clothed person [20]. Translated into food terms, that is 2.5 litres of extra milk each day. More surprisingly, an air current which is imperceptible at the conscious level has been shown to increase the heat loss of exposed body surface by 20–75%.

As already mentioned, exposure to rain, or immersion in water may increase heat loss enormously. While dry clothing insulates, wet clothing does not. Normal indoor clothing can contain 3 kg of water when wet, and if not removed, the heat needed for evaporation must emanate from the body. An extra 1,700 kcal would be required, which in some countries is equal to the average daily food intake of an adult. As an arbitrary calculation, if enough shelter is provided to prevent a person from being drenched once a week, this represents at best, the caloric equivalent of half a litre of milk a day and at worst, the difference between death from exposure and survival [20].

Direct proof of these estimates for disaster-affected populations is lacking. But that the risk of hypothermia may be substantial, even in the tropics, is illustrated by a series of 24 cases of adults with hypothermia admitted to hospital in Kampala, Uganda, between January 1970 and January 1972 [21]. Hypothermia (rectal temperature less than 35 °C) was diagnosed in all 24, and severe hypothermia (rectal temperature of 29–33 °C), in 8. This group admittedly consisted mainly of vagrants suffering from a range of diseases. However, temperatures in Kampala, which is located on the equator, are very constant, the mean minimum temperature throughout the year ranging from 16 to 18 °C.

Specific Population Groups

So far, the discussion has assumed that, for a given level of insulation, individuals face approximately equal risks from exposure. However, both children and older people have a relatively greater susceptibility to environmental exposure. In many developing countries, children under the age of 5 years may account for as much as 15% of the entire population.

In general, children are less able to tolerate environmental extremes for the reason that they are smaller and have a larger surface area relative to their body weight. A baby weighing 10 kg has a surface area of about 0.5 m², or 0.05 m²/kg of body weight. An adult of 25 years weighing 68 kg with a surface area of 1.8 m² has a surface area of 0.027 m²/kg of body weight, or about half that of the baby. A baby also loses heat more rapidly because of a lower insulation between the body surface and the air, probably due to the lower radius of curvature of the baby's body, and because of lower tissue insulation.

The LCT of a neonate is considerably higher than that of an adult; increased metabolic activity may occur at skin temperatures as high as 35–37 °C. The LCT rises as an infant gets older. Whereas exposure to alpine temperatures increases the metabolism of adults by 38–79%, it increases that of children by 72–225% [20].

Children with PEM are even less resistant to cold. The removal of a child with PEM from its normal outside environment, or from the warmth of contact with its mother, may be sufficient to precipitate hypothermia [16], even in the tropics. The most important factor in these cases is probably deficient heat production – although such children may have little subcutaneous fat – and from body wasting, a relatively large body surface area per unit of body weight.

In the rural areas of developing countries, it is not uncommon to find as many as 10% of all children in the age range 1–3 years to be suffering from some degree of PEM e.g. less than 80% weight for height compared with reference values from American children. (The weight of a measured child as a percentage of the median value of weights of wellnourished children of the same height; 80% corresponds to about 2 SD below the mean for western children). One might expect the tolerance of these children to exposure to be less than their better-fed peers.

The role of cold stress in the aetiology of PEM, and its contribution to seasonal variation in PEM prevalance and different clinical presentations, is an important but largely unstudied problem.

The Conditions to Which Populations Are Exposed after Natural Disaster

Physiological considerations alone indicate that human exposure to even quite modest environmental extremes will, if sufficiently prolonged, result in increased energy expenditure at best, and in death from hypothermia at worst. Moreover, these effects should be most severe in children and the sick, both groups which are heavily represented in disaster-affected populations in developing countries.

However, it is obvious that to obtain any estimate of the actual physiological and nutritional outcome in any specific case, it is also necessary to define the environment to which affected populations are actually exposed. Disaster-affected populations, even when faced by sudden and unexpected loss of housing, are not necessarily faced by the full risks of the environment of the area in which they live. By finding alternative shelter, windbreaks and other means, individuals may rapidly reestablish an environment for themselves quite different from the ambient environment of the area in which the disaster has occurred. This pattern of behaviour, sometimes called 'behavioural thermo-regulation', is of crucial importance in understanding the likely effect of environmental exposure on disaster victims.

Unfortunately, the record of environmental conditions faced by disaster victims is almost entirely anecdotal. Apart from a survey by *Sommer and Mosely* [22], after cyclone and storm surge in eastern Bengal in 1970, there is no other published example of systematic quantification even of housing losses after disaster, much less of a definition of shelter needs in terms of survival. However, there are sufficient observations to suggest that, within limits, disaster-affected populations are effective at rapidly reestablishing the basic 'micro-climate' needed for survival. This they achieve in two main ways: (1) by moving into undamaged buildings and (2) by building or finding temporary shelters.

Population Movements into Undamaged Buildings Within or Outside the Affected Area

Most communities have many more buildings than are required for the basic shelter of the population. Perhaps the commonest solution found to the problem of homelessness is for people to move in with friends and relatives, or to occupy schools and other public buildings.

In Nicaragua, following the 1972 earthquake which demolished much of Managua, it is estimated that about 250,000 people were made homeless. About 90% of these were taken into the homes of relatives and friends. A census taken 4 weeks after the earthquake in four outlying towns indicated that 130,000 people in these towns alone had been absorbed by extended families [8]. Three weeks later, 80,000 people still resided in these towns. Figure 3 shows the numbers of people resident in tents and emergency shelters compared with those absorbed by extended families in Masaya, a town 15 miles from Managua.

In the study by *Sommer and Mosely* [22], after the Bangladesh cyclone and storm surge of 1970, it was found that more people migrated into existing family units than in an unaffected area used as a control (fig. 4 and 'Death and Injury'). This movement was most marked in females, who

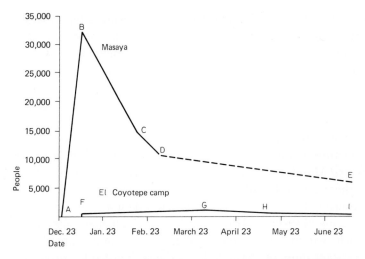

Fig. 3. Refugee population of Masaya, and population of E1 Coyotepe camp December 23 to June 23, 1973, following earthquake in Managua, Nicaragua (1973). A = earthquake; B = mid-January, approximately 32,000 refugees in Masaya, mainly living with relatives; C = official census February 15, 14,100 refugees; D = at census (10,200 people stated they would not be returning to Managua); DE = gradual drift back to Managua, rate conjectural; FI = population housed in temporary housing, E1 Coyotepe camp; F = 880 people; G = 1,300 people; H = 846 people; I = 745 people. From *Davis* [8].

showed net migration into existing families at all ages. This resulted mainly from family units who had lost their male heads, seeking the security of related families.

In Italy, after the earthquake near Naples in 1980, many people found temporary shelter by moving to cars, railway carriages and cow sheds [24].

The Building of Temporary Shelters

It has often been noted that populations made homeless by disaster are quickly able to find or build windbreaks, or to build temporary, but sometimes very adequate, shelter.

In Guatemala, after the earthquake in 1976, it was estimated that 59,000 housing units were destroyed in Guatemala City (40% of the

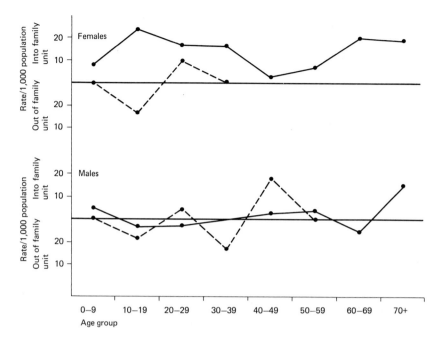

Fig. 4. Age-specific net migration rates into and out of family unit in area affected by 1970 Bengal cyclone and storm surge (——) compared with control area (- - -). From *Sommer and Mosely* [22].

housing stock), and a further 163,000 in the rural areas. In the highlands, at the season of the earthquake, the days are sunny and warm, but at night, at an altitude of 6,000 ft, temperatures can approach the freezing point.

De Ville de Goyet et al. [26] noted that the extended family system was unable to absorb all the affected population, since whole communities and entire families were often made homeless. 'Most people had lost their bedding and extra clothing under the rubble, and it took most of the first week for sufficient usable articles to be excavated. Meanwhile, the only possibility was for rough shelters, which were built immediately out of any material to hand: plastic and corrugated metal sheeting, wood, cloth and cardboard.' A steady improvement in the quality of buildings was noted. 'Cardboard was soon replaced by wood or corrugated metal before long, kitchens began to be added to the original one-room dwellings.'

According to *Davis* [9] a rough estimate suggested that in Guatemala City, 50,000 improvised dwellings were in use within 24 h of the earthquake.

The Peru earthquake of 1972 also occurred in a highland area. In one highland village, 'the improvised shelters were in poor condition; they were undoubtedly very cold at night, and would not last until the rainy season arrived. Inside the houses there was little food, few personal belongings, and sometimes only two blankets for a family of eight . . . blankets and warm clothing were needed, but there seemed to be no immediate health problem . . .' [12].

These examples are from earthquakes, where it would be expected that basic building materials could be easily salvaged, where fuel from damaged buildings might be relatively abundant, and where large numbers of buildings might be expected to survive. That death from exposure had not been observed in these instances presumably reflects its absence or rarity in populations which were dry, clothed and able to get out of the wind.

Only where people are trapped for long periods under the wreckage of houses would death from exposure be expected to occur as a consequence of earthquakes. This could happen with houses of substantial construction combined with slow and difficult rescue work. After the earthquake of November 23, 1980, in Campania and Basilicata in southern Italy, 'many dead people extracted from the rubble showed no signs of physical injury and had probably died of cold, dehydration or shock'; 'the cries of survivors who were trapped faded out after two nights of dry but cold weather, during which most had died of exposure' [1]. However, in the same earthquake, 3 newborn babies (one of whom was premature) were rescued alive from the ruins of the hospital at Sant'Angelo dei Lombardi 3 days after the earthquake; a 68-year-old man was saved 5 days after the earthquake.

A further indication of the severity of exposure risk is provided by the priorities which were set by the people themselves after some disasters. People often regard the acquisition of emergency shelter provided by relief agencies as a lower priority than guarding land and property or maintaining the integrity of the family unit.

For example, in San Martin, after the earthquake of 1976 in the Guatemalan highlands, 3,000 tents were set out by the army; 2 weeks later, only seven were occupied, despite the threats by the army to force people to live in them at gunpoint [9]. To some extent, this reluctance resulted from the feeling that the ownership of a house site, and the rubble which would be used in reconstruction was threatened by wholesale clearance. In Sicily, after the earthquake in 1968, where much of the population was living in tents and shacks, efforts to transfer children to more adequate housing were unsuccessful [13]. *Davis* [9] noted that similar attempts at 'expulsion policies' were equally unsuccessful in such diverse places as Darwin, Australia; Skopje, Yugoslavia, and the Bustee camps in Bangladesh.

One instance in which a policy of evacuation may have been more successful in preventing environmental exposure, was following the Van earthquake in eastern Turkey in 1976. This earthquake reportedly left over 50,000 people homeless [25]. *Krimgold* [15], who visited the area after the earthquake, stated that although there were delays in the immediate provision of tents, the risk of exposure was reduced by an unusually warm winter in the area and the policy adopted by the Turkish government of offering relief only to people who would move to lower and warmer altitudes. It is possible that in this area, in a normal winter, when temperatures can drop to −30 °C, the exposure risk would be substantial.

In these cases, the definition of environment is clearly insufficient even to speculate with any confidence about the more subtle metabolic effects of exposure on the population. On physiological grounds one might suppose that it would be difficult, at least for children and the elderly, to remain within the 'thermoneutral zone'. In Sicily, for example, where the typical tent for at least the first month after the earthquake of 1968 had 'a straw floor, no heat, no electricity, an inadequate number of beds . . .' [13] and where 'night temperatures were in the thirties (Farenheit)', one might suppose that this was so. Such conditions certainly might be expected to cause hypothermia in older persons living alone [18]. 2 months after the Bangladesh cyclone of 1970, 53% of the housing surveyed was 'inadequate' usually 'tiny grass huts, 3 or 4 ft high and perhaps 6 ft long' [22]. Similarly, it is difficult to believe that the conditions already described in a highland village in Peru would be other than marginal for the survival of malnourished children.

In order to find examples in which the likelihood of death from exposure could be more convincingly demonstrated, and an increased food requirement certain, it is necessary to turn to instances where all the physiological 'ingredients' necessary for exposure are present, and where the population has little immediate chance of protecting itself; that is, cases where a thin, poorly nourished and poorly clothed population is exposed to wind and wetness. Only one published case fits this description, the account by *Cohen and Ragharulu* [6] of events after the Andhra

Pradesh cyclone and storm surge disaster in southern India in 1976. Even here, however, the evidence is largely circumstantial.

On the evening of November 19, 1977, a cyclone and storm surge ranging from 3 to 7 m in depth, struck coastal Andhra Pradesh in south-eastern India. The storm surge struck on a front of about 80 km, and penetrated in some places as much as 25 km inland. Approximately 8,000–10,000 people were killed immediately, or died during the night. The population of the area are chiefly poor farmers, fishermen and their families, who are normally lightly clothed.

From a series of graphic accounts by survivors of the storm surge, it is clear that most of the deaths were from drowning, and to a smaller extent from the collapse of houses and falling trees. However, there are indications that some deaths did not occur in this way: *Cohen and Ragharulu* stated that 'survivors (and the personnel who cleared corpses) suggest that quite a few of those who were still alive after the storm might have died due to a lack of assistance, water or medical attention.' Estimates from independent agency and government sources suggest that 1–10% of those who died were alive after the cyclone and storm surge hit, but died before relief and rescue teams could reach them. Of 13 persons rescued by the Indian Air Force by helicopter from house tops and trees on the 22nd and 23rd of November, one was an elderly woman who died of exhaustion and shock before the rescue team arrived [6].

Some individuals were reported to have been stranded in tree tops for over 15 h. 'A large number died there, and corpses draped the palms in many areas of Divi and Bandar'. It was also said by survivors that 'when confronted with the realization of what had happened, many who survived the flood gave up and died during the night'. Some rescue groups claimed also to have found a number of bodies for which there was no obvious cause of death. The true cause of death will of course never be known, but environmental exposure would seem to be logical explanation.

In both the Andhra Pradesh cyclone and storm surge and the similar disaster which struck east Bengal in 1970 (see 'Death and Injury'), it was noted that a disproportionate number of the young and the old were killed. The relatively high nutritional status of children noted by *Sommer and Mosely* [22] in a survey 2 months after the east Bengal cyclone of 1971, probably resulted at least in part from a relatively high mortality of malnourished children in the disaster, and possibly also to improved food supplies to survivors.

In coastal Bangladesh, in the month of the cyclone, the mean minimum temperature was 13 °C, and wind speed 12.9 km/h [23]. It is not unreasonable to suppose that this selective mortality may have been partly due to the susceptibility of this group to exposure.

Prolonged immersion in water below body temperature from any cause would be expected to cause hypothermia and death in many individuals. *Keatinge* [14] considers that many of the 700–1,000 deaths which occur annually in coastal and inland waters of Britain, which are normally ascribed to drowning, are in fact due to hypothermia. There seems no reason to suppose that the risks from immersion after floods are any different, and every reason to think that the age groups affected would be even more prone to hypothermia than this group, made up chiefly of swimmers and seamen. *Coolidge* [7] mentions the treatment of 'exposure' in survivors of the Rapid City flood of 1972. *Bennet* [3] notes that, had the Bristol floods in England occurred in winter rather than in July, the risk of exposure in survivors who were soaked through, might have been considerable. To the best of our knowledge there are no other published accounts of exposure after floods nor of the exposure of disaster survivors to environmental conditions which might cause heat stress.

Conclusions

(1) Although most of the evidence is theoretical and circumstantial, it is probable that some disaster mortality results from environmental exposure.

(2) The risks of death from exposure after disaster are greatest in the young, the old and the sick.

(3) Death from exposure is most likely where a disaster results in the exposure of a population to windy and wet conditions. This risk is greatest in populations who are physically thin, poorly fed and poorly clothed. These conditions are most likely to be found after storm surge and floods in tropical and sub-tropical areas rather than in countries with cold climates.

(4) It is probable that the food requirements of a population are increased by environmental exposure after many types of disaster. Where these requirements are not met, an increased prevalence of malnutrition in survivors, particularly in children may result.

The practical implications of these conclusions are discussed in 'Psychological Response to Disasters'.

References

1   Alexander, D.: The earthquake of 23 November 1980 in Campania and Basilicata, southern Italy (International Disaster Institute, London 1981).

2   Ambreyses, N.: Personal communication.

3   Bennet, G.: Bristol floods 1968 – controlled survey of effects on health of local community disaster. Br. med. J. *iii:* 414–458 (1970).

4   Blum, H.F.: The solar heat load; its relationship to total heat load and its relative importance in the design of clothing. J. clin. Invest. *24:* 712–721 (1945); cited in ref. 19.

5   Boutelier, C.; Timbal, J.; Colin, J.: Echanges thermiques et réactions physiologiques à l'immersion en eau froide. Revue Med. clin. *40:* 2631–2638 (1974); cited in ref. 18.

6   Cohen, S.P.; Ragharulu, C.V.: The Andhra cyclone of 1977 (Vikas Publishing House, New Delhi 1979).

7   Coolidge, T.T.: Rapid City flood. Archs Surg. Chicago *106:* 770–772 (1973).

8   Davis, I.: Emergency shelter: in report of a seminar on emergency housing and shelter (Disasters Emergency Committee, London 1976).

9   Davis, I.: Housing and shelter provision following the earthquakes of February 4th and 6th 1976. Disasters *1:* 82–90 (1977).

10 Davis, I.: Disasters and the small dwelling (Pergamon Press, Oxford 1981).

11 Edholm, O.G.: Man – hot and cold. The Institute of Biology's studies in biology, No. 97 (Arnold, London 1978).

12 Glass, R.I.: Pishtacos in Peru. Harvard Med. Alum. Bull. *12:* 12–14 (1971).

13 Haas, J.E.: The western Sicily earthquake of 1968 (National Academy of Sciences, Washington 1969).

14 Keatinge, W.C.: Survival in cold water; the physiology and treatment of immersion hypothermia and of drowning (Blackwell, Oxford 1969); cited in ref. 18.

15 Krimgold, F.: Personal communication.

16 Lawless, J.; Lawless, M.M.: Kwashiorkor – the result of cold injury in a malnourished child? Lancet *ii:* 972–975 (1963).

17 Mount, L.E.: Adaptation to thermal environment (Arnold, London 1979).

18 Maclean, D.; Emslie-Smith, D.: Accidental hypothermia (Blackwell, Oxford 1977).

19 Newburgh, L.H.: Physiology of heat regulation and the science of clothing (Saunders, Philadelphia 1949).

20 Rivers, J.P.W.; Brown, G.A.: Physiological aspects of shelter deprivation. Disasters *3:* 20–23 (1979).

21 Saidikali, F.; Owen, R.: Hypothermia in the tropics – a review of 24 cases. Trop. geogr. Med. *26:* 265–270 (1974).

22 Sommer, A.; Mosely, W.H.: East Bengal cyclone of November 1970. Lancet *i:* 1029–1036 (1972).

23 Statistical year book of Bangladesh, 1979 (Bureau of Statistics, Government of People's Republic of Bangladesh, Dacca 1979).

24 Stephenson, R.: Personal communication.

25 UNDRO: Report of the United Nations disaster relief coordinator on the carthquake in Van Province, Turkey, November 24, 1976, report No. 003 (UNDRO, Geneva 1977).

26 Ville de Goyet, C. de; Cid, E. del; Romero, A.; Jeannee, E.; Lechat, M.: Earthquake in Guatemala – epidemiological evaluation of the relief effort. Bull. Pan. Am. Hlth Org. *10:* 95–109 (1976).

4. Food and Nutrition

Introduction

There are few published accounts of any aspect of either the food supply to populations or individuals, or other aspects of nutrition after any type of natural disaster; even fewer detail a systematic approach to the assessment or resolution of food problems faced by affected populations. Three main types of relief food distribution have been undertaken after natural disasters: (1) Small-scale food distribution of the 'coffee and biscuits' type, intended mainly as a comfort to victims rather than as a life-saving measure. (2) The distribution of supplies which simply arrive, unre-quested from abroad. In some instances this may simply be a method of getting rid of unwanted supplies with the minimum inconvenience and cost, disregarding nutritional need.[1] (3) Large-scale distribution of staple foodstuffs, either provided free or sold through commercial channels, seen as necessary for the survival of all or part of a population.

In this chapter, we are concerned mainly with the third category, specifically with evidence which points to the nature, severity and duration of the food problems which may follow natural disasters in different parts of the world. As in previous chapters, the discussion is confined to disasters

---

[1] For example, an account of the 'Nutrition Officer in Disasters' by *Gueri,* written after the experience of the Souffriere volcano and hurricane David, states that 'Relief begins to come in, of the most varied and sometimes bizarre type, from baby foods to tomato ketchup. Food distribution must start as soon as possible; but because of the large variety and small stocks of commodities sent in by governments, agencies, private organizations and individuals, food distribution is a day-to-day exercise' [15].

caused by earthquakes, floods and destructive winds; famine and famine relief have been deliberately excluded.

At first sight, this division may appear artificial, particularly as the relationship between natural disaster and famine in poor countries is often presented as one of cause and effect. Historically, many cases can be found of famine preceded by the destruction of crops and livestock by natural disasters. Most often, famine has followed drought, floods or crop disease, although a wide range of agents may be involved. For example, in 1816 a widespread crop failure in North America and Europe was caused by climatic changes following the eruption of a volcano in Java which occurred the preceding year [27].

However, the relationship between the failure of food production in a given area, and a fall in food consumption by the population is, with rare exception, more complex. The processes which connect disaster with famine and starvation involve not only questions of food production, but also the mechanisms for the redistribution of available food within populations in affected areas and among wider populations. For example, the great Bengal famine of 1943/44, which killed some 2 million people, has often been reported as resulting from crop damage from floods. However, *Sen* [24] has shown that during the famine year, the availability of food in Bengal was greater than during several previous non-famine years; starvation resulted from a sharp increase in the price of rice due to speculation and hoarding. Starvation affected mainly the landless labouring classes, fishermen and artisans who depended on the market for food.

In 1974/75, Bangladesh was affected by a famine with similar underlying causes, although mortality was much less. Part of this famine, which is metioned in this chapter, is most reasonably regarded as a direct result of floods, but as in 1943, starvation in the country at large was not the result of food shortage but of a sudden and substantial rise in food prices [23]. Many similar examples can be found, particularly from the last half of the 19th century in India, the century before that in Europe and perhaps increasingly in Africa [23].

Other societies, and particularly those living in semi-arid zones, may show a remarkable resilience in the face of crop failure and livestock loss. These societies, through long experience of drought risk, utilize a variety of systems of food storage, capital accumulation and social systems which permit rationing within wider social groups. As a result they can survive fluctuations in production which would spell starvation elsewhere, although in many areas this resilience is declining, partly as a result of increasing population pressure on the land. Further, in the last 20 or 30 years, the distribution of food after disaster has become almost routine. Although the published record of most of these relief operations is poor, it is certain that in some cases at least, famine has been averted. It is therefore fair to say that while famine is sometimes preceded by natural disaster, natural disaster has been, in recent times at least, only rarely followed by famine and the distinction is clearer than it might appear at first sight.

The following section is a summary of those few case examples available which describe the effects of natural disaster on food supply, storage, distribution and consumption. Although these examples are too few to permit making confident generalizations about the effects of disaster on food supply, they do serve to point up the major issues involved in the most common types of disaster as these affect poor countries.

Earthquake

Guatemala, February 1976

Of all natural disasters, the earthquake which struck Guatemala on February 4, 1976, has generated the most controversy about the relationship between natural disaster, food supply and the need for food distribution. Immediately after the earthquake, some 5,000 t of foodstuffs were released from stock[2] for immediate distribution, and in the following year a further 24,000 t (total value approximately $ 8 million) [12] were distributed through a variety of programmes (fig. 1). Approximately 10,000 t/annum of food aid were used on a variety of programmes prior to the earthquake year.

This programme of food distribution has come under fire for being unnecessary, and for actually hindering the recovery of the rural poor by depressing the price of staple foodstuffs, on which farmers depend for their income. While we are unable to resolve the controversy, the case is reasonably well documented and provides a good illustration of the impact of a major earthquake on the food supply of a poor country.

---

[2] Mainly United States (PL480 Title II given free to a country for free distribution) stocks [12] made up of corn, beans, wheat and oats (total 17,800 t) plus whey-soy milk powder, cooking oil and 'other', totalling 7,000 t. *Long* [17] also reported the arrival of 10 t of potatoes, tinned peaches and vegetables, wheat flour, cake mixes, sweets and even several jars of caviar.

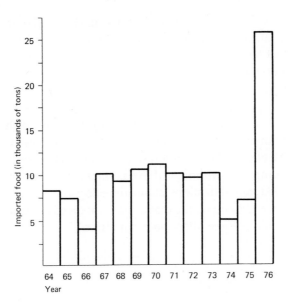

Fig. 1. Quantities of PL 480 Title II food imported to Guatemala, by year, from 1964 to 1976. Data from *Froman* et al. [12].

The earthquake affected, to a greater or lesser extent, nearly half of the 6 million people who live in the country, over an area of 40,000 km² in three main regions. The western highlands are inhabited mainly by Indians of the Quiche and Cachiquel groups and the central highlands and northeastern regions, mainly by people of Spanish or mixed descent [22]. The most severely-affected area was in the western highlands, where material damage of up to 100% and mortality as high as 21% were recorded [34]. Road communications in this area, which is mountainous and affected by landslip, were almost completely destroyed.

In the rural areas, the majority of the population live on small holdings. In a survey of San Juan Comalapa, in the highlands west of Guatemala City, *Wemys and Holt* [34] found that (of 100 families) 12% were landless, and 63% held between 1 and 10 cuerdas (1 cuerda = approximately 40 m²). Many families produce less than their food requirement and must take wage employment to buy all or a supplement to the family food supply. In Comalapa, 90% of respondents were engaged in secondary occupations, ranging from agricultural labouring (21%) and commerce (9%) to a variety of craft occupations. In a survey in 1976, *Bates* et al. [4]

found that only 3.6% of a highland population claimed to produce 75% of the household food requirement from their own land, and 27.2% produced none. The main staples grown are corn and beans [17] although wheat and oats are also produced as cash crops [5].

In Guatemala City, most of the population depend upon wage employment to obtain food. The part of the urban population most severely affected by the earthquake appear to have been slum dwellers living in shanty towns[3] built on the ravines around the city, the land most subject to landslip. The survey by *Wemys and Holt* [34] in two such settlements after the earthquake found that approximately 10% of the population was unemployed, and that average household income was reported to be around $ 40/month.

At the time of the earthquake, the staple maize harvest was complete in most areas [5] but the wheat harvest, which ripens later, was interrupted by the disaster. In Comalapa it was estimated that not more than 1% of the wheat harvest had been lost in the earthquake from landslips on the hillsides, but there was a 'pressing danger that the over-ripe wheat would begin to spill to the ground' [34]. Several observers were impressed with the lack of impact the earthquake had had upon the harvest [5, 12, 18, 34]. It is estimated that the harvest was the best in 6–7 years; official estimates suggest that maize and bean production had risen by nearly 30% over the previous year [5].

The earthquake, therefore, struck a divided country both ethnically and economically. The rural population lived on fragmented holdings too small for subsistence, and generally required cash labour to buy food and restore their houses and property; the impoverished urban population was almost entirely dependent upon the market for food. Food production appears not to have been much affected. The arguments both for and against relief food distribution revolve around the effects of the earthquake on stored food, food prices, demand and distribution.

Household Stocks in Rural Areas
Immediately following the earthquake, most observers concluded that household stores of maize and other basic grains could be salvaged from damaged houses. In Comalapa [34] and elsewhere in the highlands [5]

---

[3] The population of Guatemala City has expanded enormously in recent years. In 1966, the population was estimated at 672,094; this had increased to 1,016,118 by 1975, due mainly to migration from the rural areas [8].

people were able to salvage sufficient maize and beans from the rubble for their immediate use. *Bunch and Riddell* [5] reported that highland farmers they interviewed had lost 'virtually none' of their basic grain stocks in damaged houses, and although complete salvage of stocks took 2 weeks or so, farmers then had as much food available as they would have had in any year at that season. A survey by *Bates* et al. [4] between July 1977 and October 1978 found that of highland farmers interviewed in a formerly 'heavily damaged' highland area, only 4.3% reported the salvage of food from damaged storage, and 32.7% from undamaged storage. This implies that food may have been lost, as 'heavy damage' sometimes meant 100% destruction. The reasons for this small percentage are unclear. It may relate to a specific area, or to the long period of recall involved between the earthquake and the survey.

Marketing and Price of Staple Grains

Small farmers normally retain their maize for household consumption, only marketing if debts have to be repaid immediately after the harvest, then repurchasing later in the year [5]. Petty marketing tends to be conducted locally, whereas larger quantities are marketed directly in the urban areas.

Bunch and Riddell [5] reported that in the highland town of San Martin, those who were dependent on purchasing food found it difficult to obtain in the first few days because the town was cut off and the prices rose sharply. Some basic grains were brought in by the army, and by the end of 2 weeks the problem was solved. At this point the price of corn dropped from 7 to 5 cents/lb (15–11 cents/kg) perhaps 1 cents/lb below the estimated production cost [5]. Maize prices are reported to have remained at 5 cents/lb in highland Chimaltenango for 4–5 months after the earthquake [5]. A farmer in Chimaltenango reported losing $ 2.90/quintal after prices fell. He also reported that the fall in price was due to imported food 'especially since there were places we had always sold to that weren't buying because they had the donated food' [3].

Specific Commodities

In rural highland areas, some specific commodities were reported to be in short supply and only available at high prices in the immediate post-earthquake period. According to *Bunch and Riddell* [5], cooking oil, soap, rice, matches and sugar were in short supply; in some areas, coffee and salt were also reported to have been in short supply [17], and there was also a temporary shortage of lime (used for the preparation of maize for tortillas) [34]. These shortages appear to have resulted from breaks in communication. In San Martin, Oxfam (a British relief agency) brought in some of these commodities which not only had the effect of directly increasing supply, but also of forcing down the price of other stocks on sale in the town [5]. Cooking utensils and grinding stones were often buried or ruined, which created a problem of food preparation [34].

Labour

The harvesting of wheat creates a large seasonal demand for labour in rural areas. To harvest an acre of wheat, a small farmer is reported to require the assistance of two or three men [5]. In San Juan Comalapa, large groups of students arrived from the fourth week after the earthquake (100 on one weekend, 200 on the following weekend) from San Carlos University, to help with the harvest [34]. Elsewhere, there were serious complaints that small farmers were unable to find enough labour, because many had to spend their time standing in queues waiting for food handouts [3]. It was also reported that the price of labour rose and that some labourers were drawn off by food-for-work schemes as imported food was offered for work on clearing rubble [3].

Guatemala City

Here, there were no large stocks of food in houses and local shops had been damaged or destroyed. In the Colonia la Trinidad, a slum area, 'a system of municipal free handouts' was begun. As in the rural centres, those who survived the impact of the earthquake did not subsequently suffer dangerously from shortages of food and water, although both were rationed [34]. In the settlement of 35,000 people who had moved from their original home sites into some 6,000 makeshift shelters, it was reported that marketing had resumed shortly after the earthquake, and fresh fruit, vegetables, eggs, dry goods and firewood were on sale. 'Prices were slightly higher than in the city centre, since the vendors bought the goods at the terminal market and transported them by bus' [34]. The inhabitants of this settlement appeared to be amongst the poorest people; *Wemys and Holt* [34] reported social workers' claims of 50% unemployment in this group, although they felt this may have been an exaggeration. No pre-earthquake employment rates were given.

They also reported that many small businesses were destroyed by the earthquake, and survivors found that their customers had either moved or were no longer patronizing them because of unemployment and competition from free food distribution.

Breast Feeding

Solomons and Butte [25] who worked in Guatemala after the earthquake, reported that many women complained to them that their breast milk had dried up because of 'susto' (terror). They also say that this pattern . reportedly occurred in several communities but that normal milk-flow subsequently resumed.

The main effect of the earthquake on the food supply of the rural population appears to have been the temporary shortage for some people created by sharp but short-lived rises in market price. This was a more general problem with small consumer articles such as matches, cooking oil, soap and lime rather than staple grains. In Guatemala City, the problem for the population, at least in part, was one of supply to the area, mainly as a result of the temporary disruption of retail outlets; there was also a fall in demand owing to poverty caused by unemployment, although it is not clear to what extent this resulted from the earthquake and what extent it was a preexisting problem in that population.

It is difficult to separate the effects of the harvest, fluctuations in demand, and food distribution on the market. The low prices of staples after the earthquake were due to some extent to the bumper harvest, but were at least contributed to by food distribution[4] which reduced the normal demand. In addition, there is strong evidence that food distribution added to the labour shortage at a period of maximum agricultural labour requirement, had also created difficulties for small shopkeepers by reducing trade. In the short term, food distribution seems to have benefitted poor urban dwellers and some relief workers [25] but it is difficult to believe that there was a continuing requirement on the scale at which imports continued throughout the year[5].

Food might have been better acquired, and farmers' incomes protected, by local purchase for distribution after the first few weeks. One such scheme, which aimed to provide a floor-price for farmers, was supported by Oxfam [5].

---

[4] On the arbitrary assumption that 20% of total local food production is marketed in a year, imported food during the year after the earthquake would have increased this level by about 10%.

[5] Particularly as the Guatemalan government requested that these be discontinued as early as February 1976 [31], the same month that the earthquake occurred.

The Peru Earthquake of May 1972

This earthquake has raised many of the same issues about food as the Guatemalan earthquake. The earthquake, in which over 20,000 people were killed, affected a large and mainly mountainous area. The earthquake struck during the pre-harvest season and caused little damage to crops. In one highland village, *Glass* [13] received reports of damage to irrigation channels and crops and livestock, but this contrasted with observations of 'crop-filled fields, and fields which were intact and green. There were many rocks and boulders in the fields, but the crops still looked alive'. People were not visibly starving. *Rennie* [20], fact-finding in a remote area, also reported that 'Irrigation ditches (and so water supplies) had been patched up, the crops and livestock were unharmed . . . the people were cut off, had no shelter, light or heat and no cooking utensils. Everywhere they lacked salt, sugar and cooking oil; but everywhere they fed me with fruit.'

The major relief operation which was mounted does not seem to have been entirely necessary. *Glass* [14] remarks that 'Again, responding to a generalised disaster plan, the Americans acted to distribute food as if everyone in the valley were in immediate danger of famine – which they were not – and failed to consider the real food problems which will be forthcoming in future months . . . the Indians, not being threatened by hunger, and being unfamiliar with powdered milk, anyway, have reasonably enough decided to hoard their milk and canned goods. They will trade these for goods they really need when the roads are opened'. It seems probable that here, as in Guatemala, there were populations who genuinely benefitted from short-term food distribution, but it does not appear that a major programme of food distribution was required in rural areas.

The Van Earthquake, Eastern Turkey, November 24, 1976

This earthquake, the worst which had occurred in Turkey since 1939, killed 3,837 people and made 50,000 homeless from the partial or complete destruction of 10,081 houses. The earthquake affected mainly a pastoral population subsisting from livestock, and particuarly from sheep, although they also kept goats and a few cattle, and engaged in some cultivation. Little trade has been reported in the area [29].

The earthquake occurred at the time of the first winter snows, when families had laid in stocks for the entire winter period. Food losses reported by UNDRO [29] included the entire winter stock of many families, estimated at a total loss of 5,000 t, although it is not clear why these stocks were lost, or how they arrived at the total. Livestock losses were estimated at 15,000 head. The quantity of relief food supplied was 3,281 t, not including smaller international donations.

We have found no other useful accounts of the effects of blood supplies on earthquake-affected populations. One UNDRO [28] account mentions the destruction of fields and the loss of crops from an earthquake in Irian Jaya in 1976 (the most easterly province of Indonesia) and a subsequent food distribution programme. The salvage of considerable amounts of food was possible after the 1964 earthquake in Alaska [2], and *Haas* [16] mentions that homeless survivors of the 1968 earthquake in Sicily received no food for the first 2 days and inadequate food for 5–7 days after the earthquake. We have found no accounts for severe food shortage or starvation after any earthquake.

Cyclone, Storm Surge and Flood

The East Bengal Cyclone and Storm Surge of November 1970

The cyclone and storm surge which devastated a large part of southern Bengal in 1970 caused 240,000 deaths, but caused very few injuries to survivors. A survey conducted by *Sommer and Mosely* [26] [see also chap. 1, p. 36], 2 months after the disaster, gave detailed information on some aspects of the effects of this disaster on food supply and distribution within the area. This survey is unusual in that a carefully drawn sample and a control group were used. The population of seven unions in Gazaria thana[6] which had not been affected by the cyclone was employed as a control.

The area surveyed was that most severely affected by the cyclone, and covered approximately 2,000 square miles. It contained, before the cyclone, a population of approximately 1,700,000, of whom over 80% were farmers, 12% were fishermen, and the remainder clerks, factory workers and shopkeepers. The population of the area depends mainly upon the Aman rice crop, harvested in October and November; the cyclone struck at the time when the crop was being harvested and while 100,000 migrant labourers were living in the fields.

On the survey, information was collected on nutritional status, food consumption, agriculture, fishing and food and other relief distribution.

---

[6] A 'thana' is an administrative division with a population of between 100,000 and 200,000.

Nutritional Status

A survey of nutritional status was conducted, using the 'Quac' stick.[7] The results of this survey showed that the population of the affected area was even better nourished than the control group (5.5% $\leqslant$ 75% standard, range 3.3–7.4% in the affected area; 6.7% $\leqslant$ standard in the control area). This was attributed to the relative richness of the affected area, which is only recently settled and by the standards of rural Bangladesh, sparsely populated, and to the selective mortality caused by the flood which killed proportionately more of the weak and the sick, leaving a relatively well-nourished population behind [see chap. 1, p. 37]. *Sommer and Mosely* [26] noted that children in the affected area 'seemed to be the healthiest and best nourished we had ever seen in East Bengal'.

Relief Food and Other Relief Items

The major relief items received by victims of the disaster were food or cash; other items were said to be so few as to be unquantifiable. In the nine most severely affected thanas, from 50.5 to 100% of the population were receiving relief food, and between 2.5 and 43.9% (mean 13.9%) reported receiving over 50% of their daily requirement from this source. It was found that both the cyclone-affected population and the control group were eating a similar number of meals each day, and that both groups reported a similar frequency of consumption of fish or eggs in the week preceding the survey (affected area 84%, control area 86%). Cash relief, amounting to a total of approximately 24 million rupees, was dispensed for the purchase of seed or building materials but was found in fact to have been spent on food. At the prices then prevalent in southern Bangladesh [1], this sum would have been sufficient to buy approximately 20,000 t of rice, or to meet the annual requirement of approximately 120,000 people.

Agriculture and Fishing

Landholding in the affected area was found to be approximately 1 acre/person (0.41 hectares), considerably more than the 0.3 acres/person in the control area. At the time of the survey, 21% of the control area and 6.4% of the affected area were reported to be under cultivation; the area

---

[7] This is a simple system of comparing an individual's arm circumference with the median value for arm circumference of a well-nourished (or some other) reference population of individuals of the same height. The index is an estimate of 'thinness' and has been widely used as a nutritional indicator in periods of food shortage in poor populations [33].

planted with rice being particularly low. The reasons for this given by farmers were the salination of land, the suggestion that the land would no longer support crops, and the claim that labourers preferred free food relief to working in the fields. However, the common explanation was that the lack of cultivation was due to a lack of seeds, buffaloes and bullocks. The proportion of farmers with no draft animals ranged in different affected areas from 30 to 80% (mean 57%) by comparison with an average of 17% in the control area. On the basis of direct counts of buffaloes and bullocks owned, and the area of land worked by each farmer in the cyclone-affected area, the number of buffaloes or bullocks for each 100 acres (40.5 hectares) was calculated. This was found to be 12.8 buffaloes or bullocks/100 acres in the cyclone area; to attain the density observed in the control area, 123,000 animals and 127,000 ploughs would have been required.

Of heads-of-households, 11.1% were fishermen (control area 8.8%); 38.7% were not fishing at the time of the survey (control area 26.3%). Of these, 80% claimed not to be fishing because of a shortage of boats and nets (30% in the control area).

In this example it is probable that famine was averted by the distribution of relief food and money. As the cyclone and storm surge struck at the time of the harvest, it is reasonable to assume that losses of staple grains in fields and storage were considerable. Moreover, it may be assumed that without employment, the surviving landless labourers in the area would have had no means of support. The next example illustrates how, in a similar setting in the north of Bangladesh, famine and starvation followed a flood.

Flood and Famine in Bangladesh 1974/1975

In 1974 floods destroyed or damaged the Aus (June/July) and Aman (October/December) harvests in many riverine areas of Bangladesh. In the north of the country, erosion, rerouting of the main river channel and silting, also led to considerable loss of land [7]. Elsewhere in the country, crops were fairly normal. Total agricultural production and imports of staple grains combined were as much as in any of the preceding 4 years [1].

Landholding in Bangladesh is very unequal: overall, some 40% of the population own less than 0.5 acre of land or none at all. In some northern areas, where the river constantly erodes its banks, the landless comprise more than half of the population. They subsist by working as agricultural labourers, many moving from area to area with the harvest, through petty trade, as artisans, and in urban areas as labourers and rickshaw-pullers.

Few have reserves of cash or capital goods of any size, and many must live from day to day from their labour.

1974/75 was a famine year in Bangladesh. Estimates of total mortality due to famine range as high as 70,000 [19] but calculations based upon crude mortality suggest that the total mortality may have been two or three times higher than this [23]. Starvation affected three main groups. First, in some northern riverine areas, since agricultural labourers could not obtain work, they could not buy food [24]. Second, in some northern areas and most seriously in the remote Rowmari thana [10], poor people lost land, crops and other possessions directly from the flood. Having neither capital nor alternative occupation, they starved.[8] Third, there was an abrupt, country-wide rise in the price of staple foodstuffs which led to the starvation of many poor people in the country at large, as incomes did not keep pace with price increases. There is some evidence that this price surge was not directly related to the floods, but resulted from speculation and hoarding probably due to a depletion of government stocks, combined with an expansion in money supply; however, it is possible that hoarding was triggered by uncertainty about food supply created by early signs of starvation and out-migration from flooded areas in the north of the country [24].

Dodge [10] gives an excellent account of famine relief in Rowmari thana, a severely affected riverine area in northern Bangladesh.

Andhra Pradesh, Southern India: the Cyclone and
Storm Surge of 1977

The cyclone and storm surge which struck southern Andhra Pradesh in 1977, caused extensive damage over an area of approximately 75 by 100 miles and nearly 10,000 deaths [see chap. 1, p. 37]. Very little information is available on food problems created by the disaster. Difficulties in description are compounded by the fact that relief operations involved many different international relief groups.

As the disaster struck in the pre-harvest season, the main losses included the standing rice crop, cash and commercial crops, including bananas, tobacco, chillies, sugar, tumeric and cashew nuts, and the long-term damage to agriculture from the salination of land and the silting of

---

[8] Unusually, it is reported that many people did not attempt to migrate from their home areas to seek food elsewhere, but simply stayed and starved. Many of those who did migrate starved on the streets of Dacca and other cities [7, 19].

irrigation channels. Many of those killed and affected were landless labourers and fisherman, as well as some migrant labourers from other areas [9].

There is no complete account of food relief programmes in the affected area. Some cooked rations were distributed in the immediate post-disaster period; however, it is not clear who received the food, how much was involved, or for how long the distribution continued. An account by *Winchester* [35], who was involved in the relief operation, stated that only the few villages along roads that remained open received relief supplies. The majority of villages were cut off. However, he also reported no real food shortage, as the survivors could get to markets which were a day's walk away. Food prices rose sharply so that survivors often lacked sufficient cash to buy the necessary food. The real shortages identified by *Winchester* were matches, cooking oil and chillies; materials actually supplied included tents and skimmed milk.

Newspaper reports in the Indian national and the local press detailed a number of areas of concern [6]: the loss of livestock, a shortage of fodder, a fear of price rise at retail outlets, and the salination of land. There were calls on government to cancel loan repayments from farmers, to make credit available, to give priority to the desilting of irrigation channels for the desalination of land, and to conduct a survey to establish the extent of the salination problem.

About 30–40% of the damaged paddy is estimated to have been salvaged [6]. According to *Veeriah* [32] who was actively involved in the relief operation and, as of 1981, continued working on a development project in the area, price surges were brief, as the government 'flooded the market with food'. He also stated that the salination of the land was not a serious problem, because salt water runoff was rapid, and it did not penetrate deeply into the soil.

Cyclone in Sri Lanka, November 23, 1978

This cyclone, the most serious in the island's recorded history, caused 915 deaths from the high wind, torrential rains and floods, and caused extensive destruction of buildings. Maximum wind damage occurred in a band approximately 35 km wide, but lesser damage was done over a band 65 km wide, mainly in the eastern part of the island. Telephone and road communications were broken, mainly by falling trees, for several days and up to a week in remote areas, although convoys reached the towns of Polonnaruwa on November 25, and Batticaloa by the 26th [30].

The cyclone struck an area of the island where the principle crops are coconuts and rice, much of which is produced by extensive irrigation systems. In Balti, 60% of the coconut trees were reportedly destroyed by being broken off at ground level or uprooted. Paddies were flooded, in some cases up to 2 metres deep. Severe flash flooding in the Mahaweli, the main channel draining the eastern side of the country, caused some rice and other crops to be washed away.

The cyclone occurred at the end of November, during the planting season. Paddy from the previous harvest had already been sold and was stored in regional warehouses. The subsequently-planted rice was described as 'shocked' but was felt to have suffered little damage from the winds and flooding [30].

The high winds, rains and flooding affected food supply by damaging food that may have been stored within individual houses and portions of food stocks in warehouses, and by causing massive displacement of people who fled to safer locations [30]. Other than paddy farmers, many people in the eastern region do not grow their own food, except for coconuts which are grown in every compound. Food is not generally bought in quantity and stored, but is purchased on a daily basis, particularly by labourers paid on a daily basis.

The food problems identified and subsequently used as the basis of a cyclone handbook [21] concerned mainly distribution rather than supply: (1) Warehouses had enough stocks of rice to feed the population for 3–6 months, depending on the area. (2) Some rice stores and cooperative warehouses were damaged by the cyclone and some food stocks were exposed to heavy rains. About 50% of food stocks were considered to have been damaged by rain water. (3) The rain-soaked rice was found to be palatable if used immediately.[9] When distribution was delayed, the food spoiled in the warehouses. (4) Further stocks were in village cooperative stores, but because food was needed for nearly the entire community, the amounts were seldom adequate to meet more than 1 day's demand. (5) Some private food shops opened the day after the cyclone. (6) Some locally-grown foods, although not adequate for an extended period of time, were an important source of emergency food, particularly in rural areas. Local foods included wild manioc, sweet potatoes, bread-fruit and coconuts from fallen coconut trees.

[9] *Dynes* et al. [11] noted that after disasters in the USA, an abundance of luxury foods may become available. These are stored in freezers, and when power supplies fail must be eaten immediately.

In spite of the relatively plentiful sources of food in the area, shortages arose for the following reasons: (1) The lack of authorisation to distribute food. In the case of cooperative stores, special authorisation was required, which in some cases meant delay while someone went to the appropriate headquarters for permission. Some cases of food looting were also noted. (2) Transport from regional warehouses was delayed by the blockage of roads and shortage of vehicles.

According to an UNDRO report [30], although adequate quantities of food were available within Sri Lanka for immediate relief operations, the drain that this represented on national food stocks was such that quick replenishment from overseas was necessary. To meet part of this require-ment the World Food Programme provided 5,400 t of wheat flour and 540 t of pulses, said to represent rations for 500,000 people for 3 months (equivalent to 0.15 kg/capita/day).

The New England Floods, 1955
Whitkow [36] noted that after these floods, approximately 400 t of food were destroyed for sanitary reasons. He also noted that there was relatively little need for public feeding, as roads and communications were rapidly reopened.

There are numerous other reports available, noting that food was distributed after specific natural disasters, but no others of which we are aware which give sufficient detail to be of interest.

Conclusions

The evidence we have presented in this chapter is clearly insufficient to form the basis of more than tentative conclusions about the impact of disaster on the food supply of populations. The major point to emerge is that although some generalisations may be possible – for example between 'wet' and 'dry' disasters – each disaster presents a unique case which must be viewed in the context of the normal system by which a population produces, stores, distributes and consumes its food.

Effects on Food Availability
Within the Affected Area
Natural disaster does not always lead to a fall in per capita food avail-ability within an affected area, at least in the short term. Even where food

stocks have been damaged by rain or flood, this does not necessarily imply an immediate shortage, although it may lead to shortage after a longer period of time. Natural disaster may sometimes lead, as in Sri Lanka, to an increase in the short-term availability of some food items. Elsewhere, disaster (and particularly flood) may cause both the loss of family food stocks and other capital items necessary for an individual's survival, and without relief may lead directly to starvation.

Nutritional Status

The only examples which show a clear change in anthropometric nutritional status are those from northern Bangladesh after the 1974 floods, and after the cyclone and sea surge in the same country in 1970. The former indicated a marked increase in the prevalence of malnutrition in children, while paradoxically, the latter suggested an improvement in nutritional status as a result of disaster. There appear to have been no other attempts to obtain quantitative estimates of nutritional status after disaster.

Food Production

Food production may be affected in a number of ways, including the loss of land, the loss of standing harvests, and at least the temporary interruption of the agricultural potential of land from salination or the destruction of irrigation channels, and the loss of tools and livestock. In the few examples available, immediate reports of the effects of disaster have tended to exaggerate the impact on both crops and on future agricultural potential. Under some conditions production may also be affected by a lack of labour as this is diverted by other tasks and by the distribution of relief food.

Demand

Demand for local produce may fall as the poor lack the cash to buy food, or receive food free from imported sources. This may reduce the price of locally-produced food and create difficulties for farmers at a time when increase is required for reconstruction.

Distribution

A major disaster may temporarily disrupt short-term food distribution within an area by: (a) physically blocking roads; (b) physically damaging retail and wholsale outlets, or diverting their staff to other activities; or (c) creating demands on administration, e.g. to release government stocks, which conflict with normal procedures.

In the short term, the failure of distribution may also cause shortages of other minor food items and small consumer goods necessary to the production of a normal diet. These shortages may sometimes be more serious than the shortage of staple grains.

Price

In areas isolated by disaster from normal trade, where demand exceeds the supply of a commodity, even temporarily, prices may rise abruptly and cause shortages for anyone dependent upon the market for supply. These price surges may collapse with the reopening of communications, but occasionally (and probably only under very specific and unusual circumstances) the price rise may be sustained and carried out to affect a wider area.

However, in spite of the very tentative nature of the conclusions, it is clear that the assumption that a population affected by disaster is always in need of food distribution cannot be supported.

References

1 Alamgir, M.: Famine 1974 – The political economy of mass starvation in Bangladesh. A statistical annexe, part I (Mimeo, Bangladesh Institute of Development Studies, July 1977).

2 Alter, A.J.: Environmental health experiences in disaster. Am. J. publ. Hlth 60: 475–480 (1970).

3 Anonymous: On the receiving end – an interview. Food Monitor 7: 6–7 (1978).

4 Bates, F.L.; Farell, W.T.; Glittenberg, J.K.: Emergency food programmes following the Guatemalan earthquake of 1976. Substantive Report No. 3 Guatemalan Earthquake Study (Mimeo, University of Georgia).

5 Bunch, R.; Riddell, W.: Edited interview – The relationship between PL 480 food distribution and agricultural development (Mimeo, Antigua, Guatemala, August 1977)

6 Caldwell, N.; Clark, A.; Clayton, D.; Malhotra, K.; Reiner, D.: An analysis of Indian press coverage of the Andhra Pradesh cyclone disaster of November 1977. Disasters 3: 154–168 (1979).

7 Currie, B.: The famine syndrome; its definition for relief and rehabilitation in Bangladesh. Ecol. F. Nutr. 7: 87–98 (1978).

8 Davis, I.: Housing and shelter provision following the earthquakes of February 4 and 6, 1976. Disasters 1: 82–89 (1977).

9 Dharmaraju, P.: Emergency health and medical care in cyclone and tidal wave affected

areas of Andhra Pradesh – November 1977. Case study presented at the joint IHF/UNDRO/WHO seminar on Natural Disasters, Manila (Mimeo, March 1978).

10   Dodge, C.P.: Practical application of nutritional assessment – malnutrition in the flood area of Bangladesh, 1974. Disasters 4: 311–314 (1980).

11   Dynes, R.R.; Quarantelli, E.L.; Kreps, G.A.: A perspective on disaster planning (Mimeo, Disaster Research Center, Ohio State University, May 1980).

12   Froman, J.; Gersony, B.; Jackson, T.: General review – PL 480 food assistance in Guatemala (Mimeo, June 1977).

13   Glass, R.I.: Pishtacos in Peru. Harvard Med. Alum. Bull. 12: 12–16 (1971).

14   Glass, R.: Aid fiasco in Peru. The New Republic 14 (September 1970).

15   Gueri, M.: The role of the nutrition officer in disasters. Cajanus 13: 28–41 (1979).

16   Haas, J.E.: The western Sicily earthquake of 1968. The National Academy of Sciences for the National Academy of Engineering (Mimeo, Washington 1969).

17   Long, E.C.: Sermons in stones – some medical aspects of the earthquake in Guatemala. St. Mary's Hospital Gazette, London 83: 6–9 (1977).

18   Nash, J.E.: Quoted in the New York Times (November 6, 1977).

19   Rahaman, M.M.: The causes and effects of famine in the rural population – a report from Bangladesh. Ecol. F. Nutr. 7: 99–102 (1978).

20   Rennie, D.: After the earthquake. Lancet ii: 704–707 (1970).

21   Resstler, E.: Sri Lanka cyclone handbook (United Nations Development Programme, Office of Project Execution SRL/79/001, November 1979).

22   Romero, A.B.; Cobar, R.; Western, K.; Lopez, S.M.: Some epidemiologic features of disasters in Guatemala. Disasters 2: 39–46 (1978).

23   Seaman, J.; Holt, J.: Markets and famines in the third world. Disasters 4: 283–297 (1980).

24   Sen, A.K.: Starvation and exchange entitlements – a general approach and its application to the great Bengal famine. Cambridge J. Econ. 1: 33–59 (1977).

25   Solomons, N.W.; Butte, N.: A view of the medical and nutritional consequences of the earthquake in Guatemala. Int. H. 93: 161–169 (1978).

26   Sommer, A.; Mosely, W.H.: East Bengal cyclone of 1970 – epidemiological approach to disaster assessment. Lancet i: 1029–1036 (1972).

27   Stommel, H.; Stommel, E.: The year without a summer. Scient. Am. 240: 134–140 (1979).

28   UNDRO: Irian Jaya – report of the United Nations disaster relief co-ordinator in the earthquakes in Irian Jaya and Bali, Indonesia, June/July 1976. Rep. No. 002 (UNDRO, Geneva 1976).

29   UNDRO: Report of the United Nations disaster relief co-ordinator on the earthquake in Van Province, Turkey, November 24, 1976. Rep. No. 003 (UNDRO, Geneva 1977).

30   UNDRO: Report of the United Nations disaster relief co-ordinator on the cyclone in Sri Lanka, November 23/24 1978. Rep. No. 006 (UNDRO, Geneva 1979).

31   United States Government: Managing international disasters – Guatemala; hearings and mark-up before the sub-committee on international resources, food and energy, of the committee on international relations. House of Representatives, February 18 and March 4 1976 (US Government Printing Office, Washington 1976).

32   Veeriah: Personal communication.

33   Ville de Goyet, C., de; Seaman, J.; Geijer, U.: The management of nutritional emergencies in large populations (WHO, Geneva 1978).

34 Wemys, H.; Holt, J.: Rural centre and city slum after the Guatemala earthquake. Disasters : *1* 90–97 (1977).

35 Winchester, P.: Disaster relief operations in Andhra Pradesh, southern India, following the cyclone in November 1977. Disasters *3:* 173–177 (1979).

36 Whitkow, A.: And the waters prevailed – public health aspects of the New England flood. New Engl. J. Med. *254:* 843–846 (1956).

5. Psychological Response to Disaster

S. Leivesley

Introduction

A set of psychological responses, sometimes described as a specific 'disaster syndrome', have been regularly reported to occur after natural disasters. This chapter presents a review of the published literature on the psychological response of individuals to disaster to see if this generalization is supported by observation and if this might guide the provision of emergency services.

In an earlier review of the literature [23], some 2,000 studies were examined spanning a range of disasters from warfare to floods. Three main difficulties, however, arise in the comparison of these studies:

(1) There is wide variation in the methods of sampling and observation as well as the nomenclature used by different researchers.

(2) A range of disaster types is involved, from warfare and explosions to earthquakes and floods; these are superimposed upon societies of different social structure and economy.

(3) Different interpretations have been applied to the same data. Three main approaches to interpretation can be discerned. (i) There are the attempts to describe individuals as suffering from 'mental illness'. For the most part, these attempts have been by psychiatrists and others using an 'orthodox' terminology, i.e., that which might be found in a standard psychiatric text. Some have used the language (if not the methods) of psychoanalysis. (ii) The second approach is that taken by sociologists, of whom the main proponent has been the Disaster Research Center (DRC) which was established in 1963 at the Ohio State University in Columbus, Ohio, USA. Under the directorship of *E.L. Quarantelli* and *R.R. Dynes,*

the Center has pursued sociological studies of disasters. Sociologists have attempted to interpret individual psychological response to disaster in the wider context of society and social adjustment to crisis and to be dismissive of the 'mental health' approach. (iii) The 'social fabric' approach [38] which tends to emphasize the analysis of breakdowns in social link-ages.

These difficulties apply to a greater or lesser extent in comparing studies of disasters to all the topics covered in this book. However, in the area of psychological response, they are so intrusive as to render uninter-pretable much of the work which has been done in the field, at least from an epidemiological standpoint. For this reason the chapter has been divided into three parts. The first part is a brief critique of the methods and terminology used in some published research. The second part is a review of some published studies of individual psychological response to disaster, to give the reader an idea of the quality of available evidence. The third part is a brief review of the interpretations and conclusions reached by workers from different academic disciplines.

Methods and Nomenclature

The methods of data collection and presentation used by different authors show such enormous variation as to render comparison among many studies impossible. Indeed, in much of the literature the results are presented without any clear idea as to how they were obtained. As this problem is so fundamental to any conclusions which can be drawn from the literature, we have examined some aspects of this problem in detail.

Methods of Observation

Four main methods have been used to obtain data following natural disasters: structured questionnaires, informal interviews, second-hand interviews, i.e., of administrators and others who were involved in the disaster, and simple observations of behaviour. The information obtained in such different ways clearly cannot be considered comparable. For example, the study by *De Hoyos* [7] after the Tampico hurricane and flood disaster in 1955 used 'three types of "formal" informants: official leaders, private citizens who functioned as leaders in one or more agencies, and people in general'. After the 1974 cyclone in Darwin, Australia, *Lacey* [21] saw '56 children (at the Child Guidance Clinic) who were referred because their parents thought they had difficulties connected with the disaster. I had about 400 interviews with children and a similar number with their parents . . .' *Milne* [28] used a 237-item questionnaire covering four broad areas concerning reactions to the Darwin cyclone and the subsequent evacuation, which included questions on the pre- and post-cyclone economic and social status of the individuals interviewed. As often as not, however, we are confronted only with a bald statement as a general truth, e.g., 'various studies have uncovered basic misconceptions about human behaviour in disasters' [37].

Sampling

Very few reports attempt to define the population affected by a disaster, those eligible for admission to the study, or the sample actually interviewed or observed. For example, 'in the present study, 67 survivors of cyclone Tracy who had been evacuated to Sydney were studied by an objective test, the General Health Questionnaire, which has been found to be a reliable and valid instrument in determining non-psychotic psychological disturbance' [32]. (Approximately 35,000 of the survivors of cyclone Tracy were evacuated [31]). No mention is made of how this particular group of 67 survivors was selected. Other studies employ hospital admissions [1, 27] or people attending other social services, groups which may not be representative of the wider population.

Timing of Observations

Some authors do not identify the period at which observations were made in relationship to the disaster impact [4, 37].

Terminology

A vast number of terms have been used to describe the psychological responses of individuals to disasters. The most common terms used in the literature are shown in table I. These were selected from the review of 2,000 titles already mentioned, according to two criteria: (1) the paper had to refer to a natural disaster, and (2) only papers including original observations or reports of original observations were included. In total, over 160 different terms were found; the 25 terms cited five or more times are shown in table I. Depression is the most frequently cited term, appearing in 25 studies.

In the 60-year period to which table I refers, one might expect that the usage of many of these terms would have changed. A diagnosis of 'anxiety' in, e.g. 1945 would not necessarily reflect the same opinion as one in 1980, although even in the contemporary literature there is little more consistency in terminology. Differences in terminology, and presumably in the meaning of specific terms, are also found among observers from different academic backgrounds and from different countries. However, authors only rarely attempt to define their terms at all, and in the case of terms such as 'emotional parturition' and 'psychic numbing' one can only guess at what meaning is intended.

Some Case Examples

In this section, summaries of selected studies of the effects of disaster on individual psychological response are given. These examples are restricted to natural disasters in the interest of brevity; a complete review would easily form a book of its own.

The examples have been chosen from the past 60 years and we think give a reasonable account of the available material. However, unbiased selection from the literature is difficult, because it is possible to discern some clear changes in methodological approach over time. Much of the published material is from US sources. After World War II, the US Government sponsored research through the National Academy of Sciences National Research Council. A Committee on Disaster Studies was established by the National Research Council as a clearinghouse for information. In 1957 this was reorganized as the Disaster Research Group (DRG) and research was extended to disasters in other countries. The work of the DRG was continued by the DRC in 1963.

In the early work following World War II, observations of individual response to disaster were given prominence. This approach changed to some extent in the 1960s, when sociologists attempted to explain group behaviour within the framework of social theory. Since the mid-1970s this

Table I. Psychological response to disaster

Term used[1]	Frequency used
Depression	25
Anxiety/anxiety state	17
Apathy	11
Nightmares	11
Phobic reactions	11
Psychosomatic disorders	11
Daze	10
Confusion	8
Dependency	8
Hostility	8
Neurosis	8
Shock	8
Guilt	7
Inhibition of activity	7
Irritable	7
Sleeplessness	7
Enuresis	6
Stress	6
Denial	5
Emotional dullness	5
Fear	5
Grief	5
Hysteria	5
Pressure of speech	5
Suggestible	5
136 other terms	4 or less

[1] Based on a review by *Leivesley* [23] of 2,000 relevant studies.

methodological trend has shown signs of reversal with the reappearance of 'mental health' studies. The latest change possibly resulted from successful litigation in the USA after a dam disaster and perhaps partly from changes in US Government policy in the late 1960s which drew attention to flood plain dwellers. *White* [44] described the upsurge in disaster research after it was found that government investment in flood control works had led to an increase in national flood losses.

Earthquake, Guatemala, February 4, 1976

Hathorne [17] has written a descriptive account of his visit to Guatemala and interviews with medical personnel 3 months after the earthquake. More than 25,000 deaths had been attributed to the earthquake, and over 100,000 people were left homeless.

The author describes a number of interviews with medical personnel in different parts of the earthquake area. An interview with a psychiatrist at the San Juande Dios General Hospital is reported as follows:

'He stated that he is seeing a number of patients with severe anxiety reactions, but feels that this is to be expected in terms of the trauma in loss that people have experienced. He emphasized the fact that people did not have time to mourn the loss of loved ones by death or the loss of material possessions. He observed that people became hyperreligious in the immediate aftermath and culminating with the activities of Holy Week. He saw this as a positive activity which generally helped most people to complete their grief work and to work through their emotions of anger and guilt.'

At the Neurology Clinic at Roosevelt Hospital, on the outskirts of Guatemala City, it was reported that there had been a marked increase in 'convulsive disorders', but that 90% of the patients' symptoms were psychosomatic. Acute anxiety reactions were also noticed among 25- to 35-year olds, as well as an increase in domestic problems.

At another hospital in El Progreso, there was a 'great increase' in complaints of peptic ulcer stress syndrome or gastritis. This condition was not usually seen in rural areas of Guatemala. There were also complaints of continual fatigue, sleep disorders, and lumbago.

A doctor in Zapaca had four observations from his clinical practise following the earthquake: many cases of continuing enuresis in children aged 5–13 years, many cases of gastrointestinal difficulties normally very unusual in the Ladino community, 19 cases of menstrual difficulties, and 13 cases of postmaturity birth, i.e., labour apparently delayed due to the trauma of the earthquake.

Another informant described in *Hathorne's* study [17] was a Peace Corps volunteer in the Chimaltenango area. She reported an increase in alcoholism and that:

'there are still people who are afraid and that each time there was another tremor, and these still continue, some people react with great fear ... children are more emotional than the adults and that they cry more now than they ever did before the earthquake occurred. She has noticed that some of the older people do not eat. She said many people, especially right after the earthquake (and some still), are afraid to sleep inside ...

The author concluded from his study of the Guatemala earthquake area that there were no noticeable changes in the disease pattern seen in the Indian population after the earthquake, whereas the Ladino population showed some increase in psychiatric symptoms. There was a marked decrease in requests for mental health services during the first 4 weeks after the earthquake. After this time there was an increase over normal case loads seen at mental health facilities, primarily cases of 'reactive depression', 'acute anxiety', and 'reactive guilt'.

Earthquake, Skopje, July 26, 1963 [34]

Out of a population of 200,000, 1,070 persons died, 3,300 were injured, and four-fifths of the houses of Skopje were damaged in the earthquake. A psychiatric team was immediately sent to the area by the Institute for Mental Health at Belgrade, arriving 22 h after the earthquake. The team, which consisted of 2 psychiatrists, 1 social worker, and 2 nurses, remained for 5 days and made their own observations by gathering accounts from the inhabitants, administrative bodies, and from the reports of the public service, medical and other medical emergency teams.

The authors estimated that immediately after the earthquake, only 25% of the population were capable of giving active help, almost three-quarters manifested mild mental disturbances, and about 10% had severe mental disturbances which required special medical treatment.

'The mental disturbances we saw in Skopje accorded with the classification of *Janis and Glass:* [1] mild stuporose reactions; (2) escape reactions; (3) puerile behaviour, accompanied by increased suggestibility; (4) depressive reactions; (5) psychosomatic and vegetative disturbances, and (6) hysterical amnesias and confusional states.'

Immediately after the earthquake, instances of short-lived, severe, near-psychotic disorders were observed. 4 patients with psychosis were registered 5 days after the earthquake, although they had a previous history of treatment.

'A combination of sluggishness and apathy was the commonest reaction. In this way people succeeded in blocking most incoming stimuli and isolating themselves from a chaotic situation. Gestures in conversation were slowed, there was less initiative, and emotional reactions were shallower. Yet most people were able to look after their most important problems ... Depressive reactions appeared on the second and third days after the catastrophe. With the lessening of stupor came states of fear. At night people would dream about the catastrophe and by day they would talk about their experiences. Some children, much to the surprise of the people to whom they were evacuated, took off all the locks from the doors in one house. The favourite play of children was about the earthquake and burials. Thus, while adults were expressing their fear in words, children were expressing it through play.'

Earthquake, Managua, Nicaragua, December 22, 1972 [1]

Managua, the capital of Nicaragua, was largely destroyed by the earth-quake. 80% of the city's housing collapsed, 300,000 people were homeless, 10,000 died, and 20,000 were severely wounded. *Ahearn and Castellón* [1] undertook a longitudinal study of the psychological consequences of the disaster and compared pre- and post-earthquake admission rates to a national psychiatric hospital. The data covered all cases admitted to the hospital between 1969 and 1976, and the analysis was made within the diagnostic categories of 'mental retardation', 'cerebral organic syndrome', 'psychosis', 'neurosis', and 'personality disorder'.

The authors found that the admissions increased consistently for 3 years following the disaster, both in Managua and other regions, but that the increase was much greater in Managua, the area directly affected by the earthquake. Overall admissions after the earthquake increased by 79.7% for Managua and 51.4% for other parts of Nicaragua. Specific diagnostic categories which the authors quoted as contributing to the higher postdi-saster rates were: (1) 'cerebral organic syndrome', increase of 82.2% in Managua and 57.6% in other areas; (2) 'mental retardation', increase of 80.4% in Managua and 84.9% in other areas; (3) 'neurosis', increase of 121.4% in Managua and 101.1% in other areas; (4) 'psychosis', increase of 44.7% in Managua and 30.7% in other areas, and (5) 'personality disorder', increase of 79.4% in Managua and 140% in other areas.

It is suggested in the study that psychological and social factors contri-buted to increased admissions for mental illness:

'Devastated neighbourhoods, paucity of services, loss of one's supportive network, prob-lems of relocation, death of family or friends, and unemployment are factors of social disor-ganization which generate stress. Although disaster victims are directly vulnerable to these tensions, non-victims may also experience the pressures of posthazard disorganization'.

The authors admit in their discussion of the findings that admission rates to a psychiatric hospital do not automatically reflect the mental status of the population and that there are factors in a longitudinal study that cannot be controlled. They suggest, however, that the hospital policies and staff were constant before and after the earthquake, the system of psychiatric classification was similar, and that the hospital was the only mental health facility in the country at the time; outpatient clinics, though, were established after the earthquake. Despite acknowledgment of some of the problems in the study, the authors appear to assume a relationship between hospital admission rates and the disaster. They do not take account of possible demographic changes occurring in the population (see p. 81).

Flood, Luzerne Country, Pennsylvania, USA, June 23, 1972 [35]

Flooding affected Luzerne Country, Pennsylvania, in the wake of hurricane Agnes. Over 75,000 were dislocated and damage amounted to US $ 2 billion, but there were few fatalities. *Poulshock and Cohen* [35] undertook an analysis of the effects of the disaster on organizational responses to the needs of elderly flood victims. The elderly (aged > 60 years) made up a large proportion (26.3%) of the flood victims. 250 elderly flood victims where interviewed approximately 1 year after the flood. A major methodological problem was caused by dislocation of the population; the researchers secured names of 800 relief applicants to the Housing and Urban Development (HUD) and took a random sample from this list. The male/female ratio of the sample was 1:2, the mean age 72 years, and all respondents were white.

The major characteristic of the sample was that over 60% of respondents perceived themselves to be chronically ill or disabled. 55% of this group considered themselves to be severely ill. However, 85% were functioning adequately in their homes without assistance. At the time of the survey, 83.6% had not returned to their preflood housing; 40% had homes that were totally destroyed, and 50% had homes that were severely damaged but repairable. The authors found that:

'Despite the availablility of expanded social service agencies after the disaster, the sample group indicated a relatively minor need for classic counselling or "social work" types of services.'

The survey included a question on what the respondents perceived to be the most significant event or result of the flood:

'60 individuals answered that they experienced nervousness, fear, nightmares, tearfulness, feelings of being upset, depressed, isolated, and lonely. In addition,we had 14 responses expressing uncertainty, insecurity, worry, disorientation, and impermanence and still another 11 expressing a sense of loss of relatives either through death or separation; all of which could be indicators of some need for use of community health service.'

Flood, Rapid City, S. Dak., USA, June 9, 1972

Rapid City had a population of 42,000. The floods killed 237 people and caused US $ 100 million in property damage [3]. The study by *Hall and Landreth* [16] examined postdisaster economic and social changes in the community and for some randomly-selected families of victims. The latter were selected from 550 families temporarily housed in mobile homes by HUD. 50 families were initially selected, but 15 were dropped as they had left town – this was consistent with the community's rate of normal transience, 40% per year. Of the 35 families remaining in the sample, 24 were white, 10 were Indian, and 1 was black. The authors concluded that:

'Rapid City, as a community, did not experience a major mental health crisis after the flood. There was no rash of attempted suicides, no line of distressed victims at the door of the mental health center, and there was not even an increase in prescriptions for tranquillizers.'

The study of the families in the trailer park did, however, produce some evidence of psychological needs:

'Examination of the routinely collected data for the 35 randomly selected HUD trailer park families revealed that these families generally received substantial financial help from most of the available sources; yet, they suffered some stress in the months following the flood. This stress was not unburdened on the community via more arrests, delinquent personal property taxes, increased visits to the community mental health center, or more demands on the welfare caseworkers. The stress was generally absorbed more personally through heightened unemployment, increased school absenteeism, and more days in the hospital and more visits to the outpatient clinic by the Indian members of the sample.'

Flood, Buffalo Creek, W. Va., USA, February 26, 1972

125 people died, and nearly 5,000 were made homeless in the Buffalo Creek flood. *Lifton and Olson* [25] were retained by a law firm on a case for damages of 'psychic impairment' on behalf of over 600 people. They made five trips to Buffalo Creek between April 1973 and August 1974 and conducted 43 interviews with 22 survivors, talked to several ministers and volunteer workers in the area and consulted documents on the disaster.

They found a number of 'survivor patterns'. The first was 'death imprint' and 'death anxiety':

'The death imprint consists of memories and images of the disaster, invariably associated with death, dying, and massive destruction.

Anxiety and fear were found to be associated with images of the disaster which took on a chronic form:

'... fear so strong in many as to constitute permanent inner terror.'

The second survivor pattern was 'death guilt':

'... the survivor's sense of painful self-condemnation over having lived while others died.'

'Psychic numbing' was also observed:

'... a diminished capacity for feeling of all kinds.'

Lifton [24] gives a detailed description of 'psychic numbing' in a previous study of the survivors of Hiroshima:

'The epitome of the neurasthenic "survivor syndrome" and of psychic numbing in general is what we have referred to as the identity of the dead. We recall the guilt-saturated inner sequence of this identity (I almost died; I should have died; I did die, or at least I am not really alive, or if I am alive, it is impure of me to be so; and anything I do which affirms life is also impure and an insult to the dead, who alone are pure), and we can see now its suggestion of psychic numbing as itself a form of symbolic death.'

The fourth category of 'survivor pattern' was described as 'impaired human relationships':

'... conflict over need or nurturing as well as strong suspicion of the counterfeit.'

Finally, the authors observed the struggle for significance:

'... the significance or meaning surrounding a disaster, the capacity of survivors to give their death encounter significant inner form or formulation.'

The authors' conclusions from their research were that:

'The consistent psychological pattern in Buffalo Creek has been a sequence beyond protest or hope, coalescing into a lasting despair. Although philosophers have long emphasized the significance of despair, psychiatrists and psychoanalysts have also recently come to emphasize its clinical importance and the debilitating nature of its combination of chronic depression, unconnectedness, and hopelessness. . . . In Buffalo Creek we found despair to be especially widespread and to include a chronic form of depression and a sense that things would never change – one would never get over the disaster.'

Titchener and Kapp [40] were also retained by a legal team representing a group of survivors at Buffalo Creek. The size and composition of the evaluation teams varied with the nature of the families assigned to them. A full-sized team consisted of 1 general psychiatrist, 1 child psychiatrist, and 2 psychologists or caseworkers. A pilot study was undertaken consisting of interviews of 50 survivors in June 1973.

A court directive followed to interview all the survivor-plaintiffs which was carried out in 1974. The families were interviewed, and there were 'psychoanalytically orientated' individual interviews with each family member.

The findings showed that 2 years after the disaster, over 90% of those individuals interviewed had disabling psychiatric symptoms such as 'anxiety', 'depression', 'changes in character and lifestyle', and there were maladjustments and developmental problems in children:

'A clear pattern emerged from our evaluations and analyses. A traumatic neurotic syndrome was diagnosed in more than 80% of the survivor-plaintiffs, and changes in character structure were equally widespread. These changes, although they were attempts at readjustment, occasionally resulted in maladjustment in the social sense and always went in the direction of psychologically disabling limitations.'

Titchener and Kapp [40] found a large range of symptoms:

'Disorganization and sluggishness in thinking and decision making, difficulty in controlling emotions, transient hallucinations and delusions, anxiety, grief, despair, severe sleep disturbances and nightmares, obsessions and phobias about water, wind, rain and any other reminder that the disaster could recur, obsessive disturbances that coalesced into group phenomena, unresolved grief turning into depressive symptoms, ideation and behaviour and depressive lifestyle, somatic complaints with probable increase in the incidence of ulcer and hypertension, listless, apathy, less social behaviour, and a lack of zest for work and recreation.'

The authors also suggest that hypotheses about emotional disturbances receding quickly after a disaster are incorrect:

'Our work at Buffalo Creek suggests that this is rarely the case; the manifestations of a traumatic neurosis do not subside with the receding flood waters. The effects may seem to disappear quickly if one is not alert to the subtle covering-up behaviour of the victims of a psychic trauma.'

The authors suggest that there was a temporary ego collapse, and the ego was damaged. Reorganization of the ego took 6–24 months:

'We found a definable clinical entity characterized by a well-defined group of clinical symptoms and changes in character and lifestyle that were related to clear-cut psychopathogenic factors precipitated by the disaster. All of us have in our subconscious memory systems encounters with the various forms of dread that a disaster awakens. There need not be any preexisting neurosis for the Buffalo Creek syndrome to become disabling and chronic. All of us are susceptible to traumatic neurosis and the "death imprint".'

Henderson [18] gives a rather different viewpoint of the Buffalo Creek disaster saying that an epidemiologist would criticize the lack of use of internationally standardized instruments to identify the case rate of acute psychiatric disorder. Furthermore, *Henderson* [18] suggests:

> 'Meanwhile, we are still presented with almost useless data such as *Titchener and Kapp's* report that, 2 years after the Buffalo Creek disaster, 80% of the population – they claim – had "traumatic neurotic reactions" and were "psychically impaired" (they were therefore given US $ 6 million out of court).'

Flood, Brisbane, Australia, January 27, 1974

The Brisbane floods covered a third of the city, causing the evacuation of 8,000 people. 5 people died, and the damage was estimated at $ 178 million [31].

The Queensland Disaster Welfare Commitee was established to set up flood units offering information, short-term counselling, and support to self-help groups. The Executive Officer's Report [39] of the activities of these units describes the welfare response to the disaster and some of the psychological consequences that were observed in the flood victims. Social work staff operated in the relief centres and supervised the voluntary staff. Attempts were made to contact every household in Brisbane and Ipswich (a neighbouring city) that had experienced flooding. Contact was made with over 6,000 households. The total number of households to apply for flood relief was 7,500 but the records at some of the flood units were incomplete. Information on the flood victims was obtained from the flood units and from visits to victims' homes by social work staff or volunteers.

The social problems that were reported from these contacts fell into three categories: (1) problems predating the flood to which people were thought to have made a reasonable adjustment; (2) problems caused by the flood relating to health, personal functioning and material/financial situations, and (3) problems aggravated by the flood (i.e., preexisting problems reappearing in an acute form after the flood).

Tables II and III record the information gathered on the flood-affected households. Table II shows the nature of the needs expressed by the flood victims and the relative importance of emotional needs in relation to health, material, and other needs. Table III identifies the specific reasons for contact with welfare services in the flood area by 2,235 flood victims. The only classification of 'emotional disorders' within this study appears in the two tables.

Table II. Needs recorded after the Brisbane flood (February 1 – May 28,1974; 6,007 house-holds)

Nature	Preflood	Flood caused	Flood aggravated	Total[1]
Emotional	408	1,623	315	1,938
Health	826	307	447	754
Material	103	8,804	102	8,906
Other	165	1,068	65	1,133
Total	1,502	11,802	929	12,731

[1] Totals in this column are flood-caused needs plus flood-aggravated needs. Material needs are: financial, social, security, benefit, furniture, difficulty with house repairs; other needs include: language difficulty, need for information or referral; recorded needs include either those verbalized by the flood victims or assessed by welfare personnel at the flood units [from ref. 39].

Hurricanes and Floods, Tampico, Mexico, September 4–30, 1955 [7]

Tampico, with a population of 100,000, was struck by hurricane Gladys on September 4, hurricane Hilda on September 19, and hurricane Janet on September 30. The hurricanes and associated flooding caused an estimated 3,000 deaths, destroyed 4,800 homes, and caused major damage to 6,500 others. In the centre of the city there were 52,000 'destitute' persons isolated for 8–10 days. A further 20,000 people were isolated in buildings in the city for up to 15 days, and in the rural areas there were 25,000–30,000 isolated for 3–4 weeks.

De Hoyos [7] visited the city after the emergency had passed and made personal observations and interviews over a 5-day period. The interviews were with representatives of organizations involved in the disaster and some of the victims. 14 of the interviews were with victims who had been isolated in the central area of the city, the Plaza area. He found that this group of people had initially adopted a 'quasi holiday' mood, but that:

'Most interviewees agreed that as the disaster continued, the tension increased among those camping on the Plaza area. This tension and the emotional strain that accumulated were apparently revealed in extreme and simultaneous types of behaviour: apathy and aggressive-ness. . . . The news of people committing suicide and the news of the increasing number of victims in the disaster were very depressing. Some informants observed that the pessimistic

Table III. Reasons for flood victims' contact with welfare units after the Brisbane floods (n = 2,235)

	Pre-flood	Post-flood	Flood aggravated	Initial contact total needs (postflood plus flood aggravated)
Emotional				
Depression	38	213	24	237
Anxiety	26	203	20	223
Neurosis	16	17	13	30 (40)[1]
Psychosis	16	12	16	28
Shock	10	160	10	170
Parent/child relationship	37	19	15	34
Husband/wife relationship	43	19	23	42
Communication	40	1	7	8
Isolation	39	12	17	29
Nervous breakdown	11	21	5	26
2- or 3-generational family	19	24	11	35
Multi-family household	9	11	9	20
Preventive/supportive contact	1	201	1	202
Assessment contact	3	707	3	710
Material need	21	807	20	827
Financial need	20	799	20	819
Housing need	24	550	240	790 (574)
Health	30	22	28	50
Alcoholism	21	3	8	11
Old age/illness	101	19	56	75
Exhaustion	5	33	2	35
Chronic illness	123	10	38	48
Acute illness	21	18	21	39
Physical disability	77	6	34	40
Injury	4	20	2	22
Nutrition	4	1	1	2
Total	759	3,908	644 (428)	4,552 (4336)

From Queensland Disaster Welfare Committee; executive officer's report [39].
[1] Numbers in parentheses as given in original report, corrected to totals shown.

reactions of the people were heightened when the news of buildings collapsing were spread among them.'

After the third hurricane there was heightened aggressiveness which manifested in three near riots. *De Hoyos* [7] said that these were related to a lack of food and water and a refusal of the authorities to let people leave the area.

Tornadoes, San Angelo, Tex., USA, May 1953 and June 1954 [30]
In May 1953 a tornado caused 11 deaths, injured 150 people, destroyed 320 homes, and caused major damage to 111 others. Damage was estimated at over US $ 3 million. In June 1954 the city was again struck by high winds and hail accompanying a tornado that die not directly hit the city, but caused US $ 2.5 million damage. In the second event only 2 persons were injured.

Following the first storm, *Moore* [7] and assistants from the Department of Sociology of the University of Texas interviewed 150 families. 73% of respondents reported that 1 member of the family was suffering 'emotionally'.

After the second event, 114 representatives of the initial 150 families were reinterviewed, and, in addition, 22 intensive interviews were obtained from persons who were reported to have suffered severe emotional sequelae of one or both storms. A few of these 22 interviews were of members of families interviewed after the first tornado.

The author found that the consequences of the two tornadoes were primarily in the personalities of the residents and their relationships with others. No indicators of these problems could be found from interviews with the town's psychiatrists, pharmacists, or welfare workers, but contact with the school superintendent and the victims themselves did provide evidence of prolonged emotional consequences. Some pupils exhibited increased restlessness; there were parental requests for children to be sent home on occasions where there was a warning of a tornado. Disciplinary problems had disappeared, and an evangelical movement in the school had become popular.

From the interview schedules it was found that there were several cases of illness of seemingly emotional origin following one or both storms. Several persons reported unexplained weakness, insomnia, nightmares, loss of appetite, and general depression. 28% of respondents said they had recovered from the first storm when the second hit. One-third of the total sample reported that they still had emotional problems within their families, and about one-fifth reported both emotional and financial problems. In total, well over half of the persons admitted to emotional problems more than 1 year after the experience.

Cyclone, Darwin, Australia, December 24, 1974

Cyclone Tracy hit Darwin, an isolated city in the north of Australia, in the early hours of Christmas day. 65 people were killed, over 500 injured, and 5,000 of the city's 8,000 houses were destroyed. On the 5 days after the cyclone the authorities evacuated 34,500 of the city's 45,000 residents by road and air. A study of the social and psychological consequences of the cyclone was undertaken jointly by the Departments of Anthropology and Sociology and Social Work at the University of Queensland. *Milne* [28, 29] has described some of the consequences of the cyclone for adults and children.

The questionnaire for the study was designed with 237 items covering behaviour and attitudes in the precyclone stage, impact, postimpact emergency stage, rehabilitation, and also the perception of the organizational services before, during, and after the crisis.

Three samples of Darwin people who had experienced the cyclone were selected: (1) 'stayers', i.e., those who remained after the impact; (2) 'returned evacuees', and (3) non-returned evacuees'. All were interviewed between July and October 1975, 7–10 months after the cyclone. The sample of 'stayers' and 'returned evacuees' was drawn geographically from street maps of Darwin. As differential amounts of damage occurred over the city, the percentage of effective dwellings in each sample was finally arrived at by using a photographic survey. 'Non-returned' evacuees were selected for the study from the Brisbane area, using government departments and welfare agencies to locate them. In the samples there was an uneven distribution of sex and marital status because women and children had been evacuated from Darwin.

Milne [28, 29] found that 'maladaptation', i.e., an expression of worry about the future, was found least in 'stayers' and most often in 'nonreturned' evacuees. Increases in smoking, drinking, use of analgesics and sedatives were insignificant, except in the case of 'non-returned' evacuees.

A total of 756 adults were questioned in relation to physical and emotional disorders of households and spouses:

'Emotional disorders included anxiety and depressive states, fear of wind, sleeping difficulties, drinking too much, and hysterical and aggressive outbursts.'

The study of the incidence and persistence of complaints found that:

'The outstanding feature is the relatively large number of women (31.5%) in the non-returned evacuee sample who suffered postcyclone emotional disorders. Females in the stayers and returned evacuees samples were affected significantly less (10.7 and 12.5%). Among the non-returned evacuee males the same trend was observed, but this was not statistically significant. In fact, the percentage of emotional disturbance among the females of the non-returned evacuee group was significantly more than that among the males of that group (p< 0.01).'

It was also found that there was a strong trend for emotional complaints to persist longer than physical disorders, and this was especially the case for the 'non-returned' females.

Milne [29] investigated the effects of cyclone Tracy on Darwin children. There were 267 parents in the three groups of 'stayers', 'returned evacuees', and 'non-returned' evacuees. A pilot study revealed that a substantial proportion of parents reported abnormal fears among their children, especially when they were exposed to the sounds of strong wind and rain. Some regressive and aggressive phenomena were also noted. The types of postcyclone behavioural disturbance reported among the children included: fear of rain and wind, fear of the dark, fear of jet air-noise, clinging to mother, bed wetting, thumb sucking, temper tantrums, fighting, biting and kicking, deliberately breaking things:

'Except for fear of rain and wind, which was reported for more than a quarter of the children, the frequencies of the behaviour disturbance are generally small, and in the case of thumb sucking and the three aggressive variables, fairly negligible. None of the sex differences was significant.'

In another study, *Western and Milne* [43] developed a Disaster Impact Scale, using a sample of 200 of the completed questionnaires. They identified primary impact variables – psychological stress, physical injury, damage to dwelling, and loss of personal possessions. Secondary impact variables in the cyclone were changes in living standards and personal and social adjustment subsequent to the impact:

'... across the board one effect of the evacuation was to reinforce and increase the levels of stress and anxiety Darwin residents were already experiencing as a result of their confrontation with cyclone Tracy. Removed from familiar surroundings, with established social relations disrupted, suffering considerable physical loss, transported to areas with which they were quite unfamiliar, and housed in barrack-like quarters, it is not surprising that those who were evacuated suffered more severely than those who remained in familiar surroundings, no matter the extent of this latter group's loss.'

Parker [33] disagrees with these findings and suggests that those who experienced the greatest disaster impact were most likely to be evacuated, least likely to return, and most likely to score high on measures of psychosocial adjustment:

'I do not feel that *Western* has provided the data to support such a conclusion and it is instead conceivable that evacuation may have assisted the Darwin residents.'

Parker [33] criticizes the validity of the scales used by *Western and Milne* [43] and argues that his own research on Darwin evacuees found that they were preoccupied with escaping, and it could have been a greater stressor for them to have stayed:

'Although evacuation required the evacuees to face a relocation stressor, that stress may have been less and the readjustment period shorter than the alternative of remaining in Darwin. Certainly, the evacuation choice allowed supportive social systems over a wider area to be engaged, and the diffusion of that responsibility may have assisted the adjustment of the sample.'

67 evacuees at a Sydney reception centre were assessed with a 30-item General Health Questionnaire. *Parker* [33] says that a positive score on this questionnaire suggests a probability of the patient being a psychiatric case at that time. 58% of the group scored positively. 48% of the original group replied to the initial follow-up postal questionnaire 10 weeks after the disaster; at this time *Parker* [33] found that 41% scored positively. The final follow-up questionnaire showed that 22% (of the 20% of the original group who replied to the questionnaire) scored positively.
Parker found that:

'GHQ (General Health Questionnaire)-positive respondents at evacuation could not be distinguished from GHQ-negative respondents by age, sex, premorbid physical and psychological health, length of residency in Darwin, or severity of material losses. However, GHQ-positive respondents were significantly more likely to acknowledge a belief that they would die or be seriously injured during the cyclone. Thus, a "mortality stressor" may be conceptualized as the initial factor associated with psychological dysfunction.'

Two other sources of information on the psychological reactions of the Darwin population lend support to the arguments by *Western and Milne* [43] and *Parker* [33]. The Darwin Disaster Welfare Council Report [6] contains a large amount of raw data in the form of reports by each of the agencies in charge of receiving evacuees. These reports give evidence of some of the conditions causing stress:

'At this time, people were experiencing difficulties associated with resettlement and stemming from a sense of isolation and feelings of bewilderment. Generally they were over-whelmed by the sudden loss of home and possessions, particularly personal items which could not be replaced and which accentuated their sense of loss. The sudden loss of income also threatened their sense of security as did the immediate break-up of the family unit and sepa-ration from their husband, the latter being accompanied by lack of contact with their spouse. The majority had very strong feelings about Darwin being their home and returning at the earliest possible time. These strong feelings about the need to return created conflict in relation to working with them on resettlement plans.'

Another source of information on the effects of the evacuation is the study by *Eastwell* [9] of the long-term psychological sequelae of the cyclone:

'When interviewed in southern cities, many evacuees were found to show symptoms of "disaster fatigue", delayed anxiety reactions, depression, hysterical and psychosomatic symp-toms (such as nervous diarrhoea on the crowded aircraft). These symptoms were not reported in those remaining in Darwin, probably because of the operation of two factors. Firstly, anyone with psychological symptoms was given priority in the evacuation, and, secondly, the symptoms were suppressed by the immediacy of meaningful salvage tasks and group survival activities.'

Eastwell [9] says that in the first month after the cyclone a small number of patients was seen with dramatic symptoms – 'shaking turns', 'inability to walk', and 'mistism'. Children became highly anxious during rain and wind squalls. There were few patients needing psychiatric treat-ment for several months after the cyclone, and only a small number were treated for severe depressive reactions:

'Certainly the most striking impression of post-cyclone psychiatry was the frequency and severity of symptoms caused by alcohol. It should be mentioned that Darwin inhabitants always had a reputation for heavy drinking; the beer consumption was said to average more than fifty gallons per year for each person. Addictions to tobacco and analgesiscs were also found to be increased in patients and in the general population.'

6 months after the cyclone, when the population began to rise sharply with returning people, depressive symptoms were encountered – 'irrita-bility', 'insomnia', and 'loss of concentration'. 'Psychomotor retardation' was not usually a feature of these depressions. *Eastwell's* [9] observations of the children at this time were that:

'Disturbed children were commonly referred to suburban clinics with behavioural symptoms, night terrors and enuresis. Often their disturbance could be traced to cramped living conditions, parental alcohol excess or parental irritability. In addition, most mothers took jobs as an aid to their own adjustment. This was detrimental to some children already showing some symptoms of anxiety.'

Hailstorm, Toowoomba, Australia, January 10, 1976

A severe hailstorm damaged 5,000 of the city's 8,000 houses and was followed by cyclonic rains which lasted for 6 weeks. *Leivesley* [22] describes a welfare unit that was established by the State Government to assist with rehabilitation. This unit focused on the 3,000 pensioners living in the disaster area and offered assistance with financial, emotional, insurance, and other storm-related problems. Over 100 people were primarily assisted with emotional distress caused by the disaster. A sample survey was undertaken of the rest of the community, and it was found that people other than the pensioners showed similar emotional responses. Three types of reaction to the disaster were observed 1 month after the impact:

'The first was seen in those storm victims who were able actively to engage in the reinstatement process. They adapted to the damage of their homes, made temporary repairs where possible, contacted their insurance companies immediately for assessment, and attempted to secure tradesmen to carry out the necessary repairs ...

The second type of reaction was observed in victims who were able to function but suffered at the same time from significant emotional distress. Victims in this group also made efforts to obtain reinstatement help from their insurance companies, tradesmen and others. However, they were responding emotionally to the shock of the hailstorm's impact, the invasion of personal territory and sudden changes in their physical and social environments. The reaction was expressed in excessive hostility and anger directed towards insurance representatives, assessors, tradesmen and other people in the street who received what was defined as "preferred treatment". Also evident was an initial cognitive confusion which was still obvious 1 month after the hailstorm, when the Storm Disaster Unit was opened. This confusion acted as a defense mechanism, a buffer between the victim and the total disaster impact. The confusion meant that these victims often made their reinstatement attempts in small steps acting on one problem at a time, without understanding the long range consequences.

The third type of response was a more severe Disaster Syndrome. It was distinguished by symptoms which directly interfered with daily activities, including severe depression in the form of apathy, listlessness, limited movement within the home; agitation which appeared in unconnected disorientated attempts to alleviate stress; uncontrolled tears and expressions of sorrow over the damage done to home and garden, and incessant worry about reinstatement.'

Discussion

These case examples have been presented in order to give the reader some idea of the quality of the material available upon which conclusions may be based. They span a fair range of the published literature in terms of disaster type and of the methods used to collect and present field observations.

The results do not appear to allow any easy generalizations about the nature, severity, or duration of the psychological responses of individuals observed after natural disaster. For example, the Ladino population of Guatemala appears to have suffered at least some increase in acute anxiety reactions after the earthquake in 1976, whereas the Indian population, at least taking the few published observations at face value, appears to have been relatively spared. In Skopje, a frankly pathological psychological reaction appears to have been evident in a very large part of the population, at least for a short period after the earthquake. A similar contrast might be drawn between the observations made after the Buffalo Creek and Rapid City floods, which produced remarkably different outcomes in populations of very similar social background.

To what extent these differences are real or merely the product of biased and incomplete observation is not clear. Almost all papers omit the information which is crucial to interpretation (for example);

(1) No information is given about differences in individual reaction within or between different social groups. In those cases where information from other sources is available, it is clear that the point is important. The example from Guatemala suggests a difference in response between Indians and Ladinos (or at least a difference in the frequency of seeking help), although it does not approach the question of the services available to these two groups, which one might imagine (see p. 114) would be very different, or alternative sources of help, e.g., village practitioners, which may have been available.

(2) Only rarely is information available about the predisaster characteristics of the affected population. The results from the Brisbane floods tend to show that in at least one disaster in a 'developed' country, fully a quarter of 'emotional needs' predated the disaster. With as many as one prescription in one industrialized country for each head of population of psychotropic drugs under normal conditions [13], the point may be important in any assessment of disaster effects.

(3) In most cases there is no information on the experience of, and losses sustained by, different individuals. Are those who show the greatest reaction the bereaved? Those who have lost property? Or those subject to constant stress, e.g., in arguments as to who is responsible for the reinstatement of losses?

Three fairly distinct points of view have emerged in the literature as to the nature of individual reactions after disaster and their place in the more general scheme of social response. For convenience these may be termed – after *Quarantelli* [38] – the 'individual trauma' approach, the 'social science' approach, and the 'social fabric' approach to analysis, although there is a certain amount of overlap among the three.

The 'individual trauma' approach is perhaps the most straightforward in that it holds that some observed reactions can be taken to be 'pathological'. This may be assumed to be a self-evident fact, i.e., the individual seeks help, or help is sought on his behalf. Alternatively, it is because the reaction appears to be 'dysfunctional', i.e., to interfere with the actions which are perceived by the practitioner or patient to be in the individual's best interest.

The other two approaches hold, in general terms, that individual reactions, if interpreted in the light of general social processes, are only to a very small extent 'pathological'. They suggest that observed reactions are essentially 'functional', as a psychological readjustment to loss; a part of the process of social reorganization or a reaction to continuing stress. Proponents of these views would not argue that people are in need of 'treatment'.

The 'social science' approach, according to *Quarantelli*, [38], initially worked on empirically incorrect assumptions about severe and widespread psychological consequences for the victims of disasters. The new model which he proposed assumed that there were a variety of differential responses. Behaviour might be either functional or dysfunctional, but the general pattern of response is overwhelmingly directed towards self-preservation. The 'social fabric approach' holds that:

'... disasters have differential rather than across-the-board effects. Some of the effects are positive as well as negative; many of them are relatively surface and short in duration. The varying problems of victims are more closely related to the post-impact response than they are to the disaster impact itself.

The social fabric position does not propose that disasters have no psychological consequences. It does see little evidence of severe psychopathology on either a short- or long-term basis after a disaster ...'

For a fuller discussion see *Quarantelli* [38].

The Individual Trauma Approach

This approach is evident in most studies of disaster until the early 1960s and can be traced back to the first studies by *Prince* [36] after the Halifax ship explosion in 1917, although it is still used today. Perhaps the best-known proponent of this approach is *Wallace* [42] who first coined the term 'disaster syndrome', following a literature review and an analysis of field interviews with survivors of disaster. He describes three stages of behavioural reaction to disaster: a shock state where many survivors in the impact area are found by rescue workers in a state described as shock, daze, stupor, apathy, stunned, numbed. It may last for minutes or hours. The docile state lasts for hours or days, and uninjured and injured survivors are relatively docile and obedient, are grateful for gestures of concern, and are anxious that others be cared for first. The third state is one of euphoria marked by thankfulness for survival and intense public spirit and eagerness to work for the community's welfare. At the same time considerable complaint is apt to be directed at mass care organizations and relief services from outside the area, and charges of looting, profiteering, and general inefficiency are voiced. Many persons suffer from feelings of depression, sleeplessness, nightmares, and general 'edginess'.

The most comprehensive analysis of individual psychological trauma is the analysis by *Wolfenstein* [45] of observations on the victims of peacetime disasters collected by the Commitee on Disaster Studies. The central core of the information was tape-recorded inverviews. *Wolfenstein* described the disaster syndrome as:

> 'the state in which the person who has just undergone an extreme event appears stunned and dazed.'

Wolfenstein [45] suggests that there is likely to be more emotional disturbance following the event for those who denied the reality of the threat beforehand:

> 'The person who admits that extremely dangerous events may occur, but retains the belief that he himself will survive, is apt to emerge from danger with less disturbance.'

Another factor which, according to *Wolfenstein,* precipitates an emotional reaction is:

> 'A feeling of being abandoned probably plays a major part in the emotional distress of a disaster experience . . . The intensification of separation anxiety which a disaster produces often persists for some time after the event . . . These reactions are also related to the frequent fear of an imminent recurrence of the disaster.'

Wolfenstein [45] found that the factors involved in the disaster syndrome include the tendency to deny the event, the inhibition of emotional response, a fear of being overwhelmed by painful feelings, and intense fright reactions several days afterwards:

Table IV. Factors precipitating psychological response

---

1   Characteristics of the disaster agent [11, 12, 15, 19, 41]
2   Personality
      Denial of danger [45]
      Expectations of averting danger [19, 45]
3   Experiences during impact
      Near miss [14, 19, 20, 45]
      Separation from significant others [10–12, 45]
      Prolonged impact [15]
4   Consequences of impact
      Physical injury [42]
      Death and injury to significant others [14, 19, 42]
      Sight of mangled bodies [2, 12, 14]
      Destruction of personal property [11, 42]
      Extent of damage [11, 12, 41]

'Since the disaster victim has been forced to take in more than he can for the moment assimilate, his energies become engrossed in the task of mastering, of gradually inuring himself to the sudden and terrible experience. With this preoccupation there is a resistance to taking in any more stimuli. The organism has been flooded with stimuli; it has not the capacity to accept more for the time being. Hence, the insensitivity of the disaster victim to what is going on around him.'

Wolfenstein [45] further suggests that the combination of emotional dullness, unresponsiveness to outer stimulation, and inhibition of activity resembles the clinical syndrome of depression. As it is a response to an exceptional situation, it is likely to be temporary, and those who are unable to recover are likely to have a preexisting emotional disturbance.

Table IV shows in summary form the factors which have been identified by different researchers as being related to observed psychological responses in individuals after disaster. All of these researchers have taken the 'individual trauma' approach.

The Reported Incidence of Disaster Syndrome

A number of different estimates of the incidence of a disaster syndrome appear in the literature. *Fritz and Marks* [12] report that from the NORC studies of survivors of 70 different disasters 14% were shocked and dazed immediately after impact, 45% were agitated, 6% highly agitated, and 8% calm. The observations by *Popovic and Petrovic* [34] from the Skopje earthquake suggest that 10% of the survivors immediately after impact had a severe mental disturbance and that 20–25% recovered quickly and reacted appropriately. The study by *Milne* [28] of the Darwin cyclone shows that 7–10 months after the impact, 18.6% of adult survivors were experiencing emotional reactions. The Brisbane flood research [38] which covered all flooded housholds found that 9% of the population were suffering from emotional problems following the flood. The study by *Leivesley* [22] of hailstorm victims who used a welfare unit service found that 16% of these victims had severe emotional problems. In the study by *Poulshock and Cohen* [35] of aged victims who applied for welfare assistance in the United States following a disaster 33% were found to have an emotional disturbance. The Buffalo Creek study by *Titchener and Kapp* [40] reports that 80% of survivors had 'traumatic neurotic symptoms'.

The interpretation of these figures, though, is subject to the reservations mentioned about methods of data collection.

'Social' Approaches to Analysis

The 'social science' and 'social fabric' approaches to analysis are also the subject of a large (and mostly theoretical) literature. A discussion of this theoretical analysis is beyond the scope of this book, but it is of clear relevance to the discussion of 'disaster syndrome' in that it tends to paint an almost entirely contrasting picture of the behaviour of individuals and groups after disaster.

This literature is open to many of the criticisms previously levelled in this chapter, but also to two others. First, many authors have reported observations which they have generalized to the 'whole community' without defining the observed population or estimating how it related to the population at large. Second, many sociological studies, and perhaps particularly those undertaken since the 1960s (although there are some exceptions before then), tend to present results directly in the context of sociological theory, such that it is difficult for the reader to separate the two.

In the following section, a brief summary is presented, based heavily upon a study by *Dynes* et al. [8] of the responses observed in groups of individuals after disaster. These observations are based on over 300 studies made by the DRC, mainly in the United States. Although there are fewer observations of group behaviour after major natural disasters in poorer countries, there is some indirect evidence from much of the nonpsychological literature to suggest that these responses are, in general terms at least, often observed after disasters.

Group Behaviour after Disaster

Panic and Flight. If the word 'panic' is taken to mean the flight of an individual without consideration for others, then panic behaviour during or after natural disaster appears to be very rare. Although some small-scale examples of panic after disaster have been recorded, it has been found by the DRC that, in general, people will often deliberately stay in a threatening situation rather than leave it. Flight from danger when it does occur appears to be the result of definite decisions made by individuals and groups, after weighing up the alternative open to them. Population movements, when they do occur, are relatively orderly and far from the pictures conjured up by media reporting, e.g., 'population flees quake city'. *Dynes* et al. [8] give the example of hurricane Carla in 1961, where more than half a million people left coastal areas of Texas and Louisiana. In spite of a clearly recognized threat, an intensive warning campaign, and more than 4 days of warning, over half the population remained in their home areas.

From the general literature on disaster, it is difficult to find reliable reports of large-scale population movement before, during, or after disaster without a convincing explanation as to why a population should have chosen this course of action, e.g., the movement of the homeless to relatives within Managua (see p. 81), or escape or evacuation from floods. Although poorly documented, it has been regularly reported that poor people, at least in much of the Indian subcontinent, actively resist attempts to evacuate them from danger, until all hope of saving material possessions has gone. *Dynes* et al. [8] wrote:

'Just as the panic image of disaster behaviour is generally incorrect, so is the view that disasters leave victims dazed and disorientated. People are not immobilized by even the most catastrophic of events, nor are they devoid of initiative or passively dependent, or expect that relief workers will take care of their needs.'

In general, disaster victims act in an active manner and do not wait for assistance from outsiders; on a large scale they show considerable personal initiative and a pattern of self and informal mutual self-help. Of the many examples which could be cited, only one will be given, from after the 1976 Guatemala earthquake [26]:

'... from the earliest hours after the earthquake, the amount of teamwork accomplished and the number of volunteer groups set up and organized were truly amazing. The first sunlight found the citizens cleaning the streets, removing the debris from falling buildings and helping their neighbours, friends and fellow citizens to carry away the wounded and evacuate the dead. Civilian patrols organized immediately established car pools with their private cars to transport the wounded, provided substantial assistance in keeping order and forming queues of people waiting to receive food and medical supplies. Debris removal began at once, as did the cleaning of streets and local roads and highways to allow the rescue patrols to come in.'

Antisocial Behavior. Antisocial behaviour is rare; it is often assumed that large-scale looting and antisocial behaviour are common after disaster. Although the DRC studies have tended to show that many survivors of disaster express concern about looting, there are few confirmed cases of looting actually occurring. Obviously, this depends to some extent upon the exact definition applied to the term; cases such as the 'looting' of food after the Sri Lanka cyclone (see p. 104) appear to be explicable in terms of hunger rather than attempts of a population to take advantage of disruption for personal gain. Examples such as the Managua earthquake, when gunshot wounds were common, appear to be rare (see p. 44).

From the DRC findings, *Quarantelli* [37] has consistently argued that:

'. . . the "disaster syndrome" appears only in the more traumatic kinds of disaster, is confined to the post-impact period, and is of short duration (its initial stage seldom enduring more than minutes or hours). More important, the reaction does not occur on a large scale.'

Conclusions

(1) There is a fairly regularly-observed pattern of individual psychological responses observed in survivors of disasters. There is some evidence to suggest that the syndrome described by *Wallace* [41, 42] may provide a reasonable description at least of a proportion of the psychological responses observed after disaster.

(2) The specific nature and pattern of these symptoms is poorly defined and varies with specific conditions. It seems doubtful if sufficient evidence exists to suggest that these form a specific 'disaster syndrome'. An equally plausible suggestion is that each individual shows a response appropriate to his or her own individual circumstances and that the responses described after disaster may be very similar to those observed after other overwhelming personal crises. A 'disaster syndrome' may describe only a large number of these individual reactions all occurring at roughly the same time.

(3) Although the published evidence is weak, it does appear that this 'syndrome' is generally observed in only a minority of individuals, is often

short-lived, and does not interfere to any great extent with individual or group efforts at recovery. Where individuals are exposed to continuing stress, this may manifest itself in continuing complaints of anxiety, insomnia, and other symptoms.

(4) There does not seem to be adequate evidence to suggest that an expansion of formal psychiatric services after disaster would be either practical or of any clear benefit to survivors. (Some authors have proposed that this is necessary; see for example ref. 5.) If it is accepted that most observations are explicable in terms of reaction to loss and the stresses involved in reinstatement of property, it would be more logical to divert resources towards meeting individual material needs and personal social problems and to avoid actions such as evacuation which may cause stress.

(5) Although there are particular difficulties in observation and measurement in this area, we do feel a attempt should be made to more clearly define terms and so apply standard methodological procedures in sampling and presentation of data; if this were done, it would help to clarify the relationship between disaster and psychological and social response.

References

1   Ahearn, F.L.; Castellón, S.R.: Comparison of pre- and post-disaster admission rates to the Nicaragua National Psychiatric Hospital 1969–1976 (Mimeo, 1976).

2   Anderson, J.W.: Cultural adaptation to threatened disaster. Hum. Org. *27:* 298–307 (1968).

3   Atlanta Public Health Service, Field Services Branch Epidemiology Program: Flood disaster, Rapid City, South Dakota (Mimeo, 1972).

4   Church, J.S.: The Buffalo Creek disaster; extent and range of emotional and/or behavioural problems. Omega *5:* 61–63 (1974).

5   Cohen, R.E.; Ahearn, F.L., Jr.: Handbook for mental health care of disaster victims (Johns Hopkins University Press, Baltimore 1980).

6   Darwin Disaster Welfare Council: Final report (Mimeo, 1976).

7   De Hoyos, A.: The Tampico disaster; a report to the committee on disaster studies, National Research Council, Michigan State University Department of Sociology and Anthropology (Social Research Service, Mimeo 1956).

8   Dynes, R.R.; Quarantelli, E.L.; Kreps, G.A.: A perspective on disaster planning. Report Ser. 11 (Disaster Research Center, Ohio State University, Columbus 1980).

9   Eastwell, D.: Psycho-social sequelae of cyclone 'Tracy'. Proc. Medical Disaster seminar, pp. 10–19 (National Emergency Services College, Macedon 1977).

10 Friedman, P.; Linn, L.: Some psychiatric notes on the Andrea Doria disaster. Am. J. Psychiat. *114:* 426–432 (1957).

11   Fritz, C.E.: Disasters compared in six American communities. Hum. Org. *16:* 6–9
      (1957).
12   Fritz, C.; Marks, E.S.: The NORC studies of human behaviour in disaster. J. soc. Issues
      10: 26–41 (1954).
13   Fry, J.: A new approach to medicine. Principles and priorities in health care (MIT Press,
      Lancaster 1978).
14   George, A.: Emotional stress and air war. A lecture given at the Air War College, Air
      University (Rand Corporation, Santa Monica 1952).
15   Glass, A.J.: Psychological problems in nuclear warfare. Am. J. Nursing *57:* 1428–1431
      (1957).
16   Hall, P.S.; Landreth, P.W.: Assessing some long-term consequences of a natural disaster.
      Mass Emerg. *1:* 55–61 (1975).
17   Hathorne, B.C.: Report – Guatemala, May 11–21, 1976 (unpublished report to USAID,
      1976).
18   Henderson, A.S.: Disaster and social bonds. Disaster Behaviour Seminar, pp. 10–18
      (National Emergency Services College, Macedon 1977).
19   Janis, I.L.: Problems of theory in the analysis of stress behaviour. J. soc. Issues *10:* 12–24
      (1954).
20   Janis, I.L.: Psychological effects of warnings; in Baker, Chapman, Man and society in
      disaster, pp. 55–92 (Basic Books, New York 1962).
21   Lacey, G.N.: Observations on Aberfan. J. psychosom. Res. *16:* 257–260 (1972).
22   Leivesley, S.: Toowoomba; the role of an Australian disaster unit. Disasters *1:* 315–322
      (1977).
23   Leivesley, S.: A study of disasters and the welfare planning response in Australia and the
      United Kingdom; unpublished thesis, University of London (1979).
24   Lifton, R.J.: Death in life – the survivors of Hiroshima (Weidenfeld & Nicholson,
      London (1968).
25   Lifton, R.J.; Oson, E.: The human meaning of total disaster. The Buffalo Creek expe-
      rience. Psychiatry *39:* 1–18 (1976).
26   McDonald, R.K.: Earthquake disaster in Guatemala. Joint IHS/UNDRO/WHO
      Seminar on Natural Disaster, Manila (Mimeo, 1977).
27   Menninger, W.C.: Psychological reactions in an emergency (flood). Am. J. Psychiat. *109:*
      128–130 (1952).
28   Milne, G.: Cyclone Tracy, I. Some consequences of the evacuation of adult victims.
      Aust. J. Psychol. *4:* 39–54 (1977a).
29   Milne, G.: Cyclone Tracy. II. The effects on Darwin children. Aust. J. Psychol. *4:* 55–62
      (1977b).
30   Moore, H.E.: Some emotional concomitants of disaster. Ment. Hyg., Lond. *42:* 45–50
      (1958).
31   Natural Disasters Organization: Darwin disaster; cyclone Tracy. Report by the Director
      General Natural Disasters Organization on the relief operations December
      25–January 3, 1975 (Australian Government Publishing Service, Canberra 1975).
32   Parker, G.: Psychological disturbance in Darwin evacuees following cyclone Tracy.
      Med. J. Aust. *24:* 650–652 (1975).
33   Parker, G.: Identification, triage and management of those at risk. Disaster Behaviour
      Seminar, pp. 36–46 (National Emergency Services College, Macedon 1977).
34   Popovic, M.; Pretrovic, D.: After the earthquake. Lancet *ii:* 1169–1171 (1964).

35   Poulshock, S.W.; Cohen, E.S.: The elderly in the aftermath of a disaster. Gerontologist
     6: 357–361 (1975).
36   Prince, S.H.: Catastrophe and social change; Faculty of Political Science of Columbia
     University, in Studies in history, economics and public law, vol. 94, No. 1 (AMS Press,
     New York 1920).
37   Quarantelli, E.L.: Images of withdrawal behaviour in disasters. Some basic misconcep-
     tions. Soc. Probl. *8:* 68–79 (1960).
38   Quarantelli, E.L.: The consequences of disasters for mental health. Conflicting views.
     Preliminary paper No. 62 (Disaster Research Center, Ohio State University, Columbus
     1979).
39   Queensland Disaster Welfare Committee: Executive Officer's report (Mimeo, 1974).
40   Titchener, J.L.; Kapp, F.T.: Family and character change at Buffalo Creek. Am. J.
     Psychiat. *133:* 295–299 (1976).
41   Wallace, A.F.C.: Human behaviour in extreme situations. A study of the literature and
     suggestions for further research. Disaster study No. 1, Committee on Disaster Studies
     (National Academy of Sciences/National Research Council, Washington 1956).
42   Wallace, A.F.C.: Mazeway disintegration. The individual's perception of socio-cultural
     disorganization. Hum. Org. *16:* 23–27 (1957).
43   Western, J.S.; Milne, G.: Some social effects of a natural hazard: Darwin residents and
     cyclone Tracy. Symp. on Natural Hazards in Australia (Australian Academy of Science,
     Canberra, unpublished).
44   White, G.F.: Natural hazards research: concepts, methods, and policy implications; in
     White, Natural hazards: local, national, global (Oxford University Press, Oxford 1974).
45   Wolfenstein, M.: Disaster: a psychological essay (Routeledge & Kegan, London 1957).

6. The Practical Application of Epidemiological Methods to Disasters

Introduction

To date, the 'epidemiology of disasters' has found three practical applications, all to disaster relief. The first, discussed at length in this chapter, arises from the approach taken in this book: that is, the classification of observations of the effects of disasters on the health of populations. It is possible to make sufficiently reliable generalizations about the effects of disasters for them to be used as the basis for relief planning and immediate relief action, before detailed information is available about the needs of an affected population. The second application of epidemiological methods to relief is the use of surveys and other techniques for information collection which, although as yet little used, has been shown to be a practical method of assessing the needs of disaster-affected populations. The third, a now well-established application which has been fully discussed [see chap. 2, Appendix], is the surveillance and control of communicable disease and other health hazards after disasters.

Detailed studies of the relationships between disaster, damage, the location of individuals at the time of the impact and mortality and injury, may have considerable potential for improving the quality of warnings given before disasters, and may also contribute to the search for low-cost methods of hazard reduction associated with traditional housing methods in earthquake-prone countries. This approach has been tried in only three studies to date [3, 10, 11], from which, as yet, few conclusions can be drawn. Two of these studies are described earlier [chap. 1, pp. 16, 30].

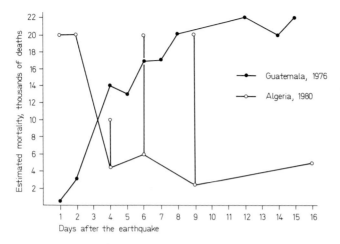

Fig. 1. Estimates of mortality on various days after the 1976 Guatemala earthquake and after the 1980 earthquake at El Asnam, Algeria. Vertical lines connect two estimates on the same day. Data from the London Times and Guardian newspapers.

Applications to Disaster Relief

Disaster Relief as a Problem of Information

With the speed and wide distribution of modern communications, the fact that a disaster has occurred is usually known to the outside world from within minutes to at most hours of the impact. However, because of the wide areas which may be affected, variations in effects within the area and the disruption of local communications, accurate information about the effects of a disaster and the needs of survivors is often not available for a period of days or weeks. Relief administrators, both within the affected area and abroad are faced with a dilemma. On the one hand, it is perceived that urgent and massive action is required if lives are to be saved: on the other, little or no information is usually available as to the immediate needs of the survivors or the resources already available within and adjacent to the affected area.

The information that is available immediately after a disaster is often highly misleading. For example, figure 1 shows estimates of mortality after two major earthquakes, in Guatemala in 1976, and at El Asnam, Algeria in 1980. Both of these earthquakes occurred in areas with good external communications. Nevertheless, it was not for several days after each disaster that the true scale of mortality became evident. It may be imagined, given the confusion after a major disaster, that these examples are not unusual. *Quarentelli* [22] has even gone so far as to suggest a 'rule' that the excess of rumoured over registered deaths increases with the distance of the disaster from the capital city. Accurate information of more use to relief planning than mortality, such as the location and number of the injured, the condition of hospitals and the location of drug stocks is usually entirely lacking.

In practise, the immediate relief response to reports of a major natural disaster has often been described as a 'convergence' of relief material and personnel on the affected area. A major relief operation in a developing country may now involve assistance from hundreds of relief organizations[1]. Enormous quantities and values of relief may be supplied, often in

---

[1] International disaster relief derives from four main sources: (1) direct government-to-government aid. The principal donors are western governments, although contributions are also made between developing countries, particularly where these share a common experience of disaster, e.g., Central American states after earthquakes; (2) the nongovernment agencies. The larger western agencies are well known, but there are also many smaller agencies involved in relief (these are estimated to number over 400 in the US alone [19]). The Red Cross occupies a special position in that it is represented by member societies in every country; (3) the United Nations agencies. The main agencies concerned with relief are the Office of the United Nations Disaster Relief Coordinator (UNDRO); the World Health Organization, including the Pan-American Health Organization; the World Food Programme of the UN Food and Agriculture Organization, and the UN Childrens Fund; (4) less visible, but often very substantial flows of assistance may pass directly from individuals to people in the affected area, particularly when there are strong ethnic links, e.g., from people of Latin American, Asian and Mediterranean stock resident in North America and Europe to individuals in their home areas. Individuals may also travel independently to the scene of disaster to offer assistance. *Locally,* the capacity of countries to organize relief varies widely. In most countries disaster relief will engage the army and other military forces, the police, fire brigade and other civil organizations. Several countries which suffer regularly from disasters have well-organized systems for emergency relief, e.g., Turkey, the Philippines. In both industrialized and developing countries, locally based nongovernment agencies may also be involved, e.g., approximately 70 Indian organizations were involved in relief after the 1977 cyclone disaster in Andhra Pradesh, southern India [5].

Generally speaking, the richer countries tend to rely on their own organizations and resources for relief: the developing countries, in addition to locally organized relief may also receive international assistance. However, in any particular case, the number and sources of assistance depends upon a complex interaction of factors, including not only humanitarian considerations but also the amount of media coverage given (which influences public perception and therefore the resources available), the historical and political links between donor and recipient and other factors unrelated to the needs of the country concerned.

the absence of any real indication of need. Shelter, clothing, drugs, vaccines, medical personnel and food are supplied on the assumption that they will be required[2]. Very little is known about the value of this relief to survivors, as almost no evaluation of relief work has ever been conducted[3]. Observers have repeatedly been struck by the supply of goods which are irrelevant to the needs of survivors; the over- and undersupply of goods which are required; goods which are poorly labelled, and the vast over-supply of goods leading to congestion at ports and impeding sorting and delivery to places in need [1, 9, 12, 36].

It is widely recognized that there are problems with the effective and efficient supply of international relief after disasters. Some steps and many suggestions have been made to overcome these, mostly emphasizing the improved coordination of assistance, e.g., the creation of the Office of the United Nations Disaster Relief Coordinator, or the speed of relief response. For example, it has been suggested that standing 'disaster forces' should be created in the industrialized countries, ready to fly to disaster areas in the developing countries at short notice; that satellites and other advanced communications methods should be employed; and that relief supplies should be stockpiled in disaster-prone countries or regions [12,

[2] Because of the large number of organizations which may be involved in relief, and the lack of centralized record-keeping, very little is known about the quantities of relief material despatched after disasters. Over 100 tons of drugs were received in Guatemala after the 1976 earthquake [36], and over 3,000 tons of clothing after the 1980 earthquake in southern Italy [1]. Table I sets out the total value of emergency relief supplied after several recent major disasters, as reported to the Office of the United Nations Disaster Relief Coordinator (UNDRO). As reporting to UNDRO is voluntary, the table may underestimate, possibly by a considerable amount, the total value of relief supplied in each case. It is widely believed that the size of international response to a disaster is primarily determined by the total estimated mortality, rather than the number of the injured, the economic loss sustained or other measure of the severity of the impact. Some support for this view is given by table 1, in which the total value of assistance is correlated with the total mortality ($r = 0.78$, $p < 0.01$), but not with homelessness, the only other variable for which relatively complete data are given ($r = -0.12$, $p > 0.05$).

[3] An exception to this statement is the provision of emergency shelter which has been very fully evaluated and clear policy guidelines issued [35]. The few published accounts of locally organized relief in the developing countries where international assistance has not been supplied [2, 8, 13] suggest that this may be, within the resources available, as effective and efficient as some relief response in the industrialized countries. It may also be noted that some international agencies have progressively modified their policies in the light of accumulating knowledge about the effects of disasters [e.g. 20]. Some interesting new approaches to relief have also been tried [e.g. chap. 4, p. 96].

Table I. Mortality, homelessness and the value of international emergency assistance after nine disasters [data from UNDRO, 26–34]

Disaster	Number of deaths	Number of homeless	Value of assistance, US$
Earthquake			
Indonesia, July 1981	993	250,000	1,551,694
Turkey, November 1976	3,837	50,000	29,986,993
Iran, July 1981	1,000	30,000–50,000	770,420
Floods			
Mozambique, February 1977	300	31,900	4,339,513
Jamaica, June 1979	40	35,000–40,000	5,493,830
Cyclone			
Oman, June 1977	105	no data	14,992,920
Sri Lanka, November 1978	915	100,000	7,859,398
Dominica, August 1979	40	no data	5,525,757
Dominican Republic, August/September 1979	2,000	125,000	22,258,815

16]. However, few observers have questioned the basic premises which underly much of the current international response to disasters: that major disasters always create needs for a wide range and large quantity of relief material, and that when a disaster has occurred in a developing country, these needs must be met from abroad.

In the following section, a more logical approach to the provision of disaster relief is suggested. This approach is divided into two parts: (1) An emergency relief response which is based upon more realistic assumptions about the immediate needs of survivors after different types of disasters, the period during which these needs must be met, and the probable effectiveness of the local relief response. Experience suggests that typically, this phase of a relief operation after a major disaster in a developing country will last for 3–7 days. (2) Beginning at a rather later time, but in parallel with the emergency response, further relief needs should be determined by the collection of information about the needs of survivors. From the first few days after most disasters, information is required to define the needs for the rescue and treatment of the injured, to improve the quality of temporary housing, to repair public utilities, to improve food supply, and to identify and control outbreaks of communicable disease. In many cases, information collection is required for months or years after the disaster to guide the process of reconstruction.

The following discussion has been directed towards the problem of relief response after a major disaster in a developing country, as it is under these circumstances that the main lessons of 'disaster epidemiology' are currently to be learned. However, it may be noted that: (1) essentially the same approach can be applied to the provision of relief after any disaster in any country; (2) the first part of the discussion – the experience of the effects of disasters on health – can also be used as the basis of planning for emergency relief. In any specific disaster-prone area, where the type or types of disaster can be anticipated, and more information is available on the types of housing, the location of medical services, drug stocks and other relevant factors, it is usually possible to make much more specific statements about the relief needs which may arise than are given here.

The discussion has also been limited to those conclusions which arise directly from the evidence presented in the main part of the book. No mention is made of relief techniques, e.g. specialized rescue techniques, the organization of emergency medical services, or the assessment of nutritional status, for which good accounts are already available [20, 21, 35, 39, 40].

Relief Response during the Emergency Period

Death and Injury: Search and Rescue and the Provision of Emergency Medical Care and Supplies

Clearly, the need to provide organized assistance for the rescue and treatment of casualties after a disaster will depend upon the location of the survivors, and the number and types of injuries which have occurred. The need to provide immediate assistance from international sources will depend upon the adequacy of the local response from the survivors themselves and from hospitals and other organizations within, and adjacent to, the affected area. Observations of disasters have shown that:

(1) While mortality from any disaster may fall within a wide range, very high mortality, i.e., up to hundreds of thousands of deaths, is likely to result only from earthquakes, storm-surge and other types of violent flooding. Other floods, tornadoes and cyclone uncomplicated by flooding tend to cause relatively modest mortality, i.e. hundreds of deaths.

(2) The relationship between mortality and the number of injured

Table II. Patterns of mortality and injury after natural disasters

Potential mortality	Deaths exceed injuries	Injuries exceed deaths
High (up to hundreds of thousands)	storm-surge, tsunami, flash floods	earthquake
Low (up to thousands)	floods	tornado, cyclone (without floods)

survivors is not direct, but depends upon the type of disaster. Injured survivors are likely to exceed the number of dead only after earthquake, tornado and cyclone. Very large numbers of injured, i.e. several thousand or more, are likely to result only from a major earthquake. These two points are summarized in table II.

(3) After any type of disaster, only 5–10% of injuries will be severe, i.e., requiring inpatient care.

(4) Some useful statements can be made about the types of injuries which will result from earthquakes and tornadoes [see chap. 1]. After major earthquakes, the bulk of serious injuries will be made up of fractures with a proportion of soft tissue and internal injuries and burns.

(5) There is no evidence to suggest that during the first few days after disasters the incidence of other (i.e. nontraumatic) disease will increase. Under some conditions, the number of presentations at medical facilities for reasons other than trauma will fall.

(6) In those few cases for which information is available, the bulk of acute medical care has been completed within 5 days of the disaster.

(7) Although there are few published examples of the reactions of survivors within disaster-affected areas, particularly in the developing countries, current evidence suggests that the majority will behave in a rational and effective manner from the first minutes after the disaster, and that survivors will become rapidly more organized with time. In areas where rescue is possible without organized assistance, e.g. the rescue of survivors from the rubble of collapsed houses, most such activities will be conducted by the survivors themselves. Where medical facilities are accessible, the survivors will also transport the injured there. Current evidence suggests that disasters tend to favor the survival of adults in the most economically active age groups, particularly the survival of adult men.

(8) Very little is known about the length of survival of the injured where lack of assistance with rescue, services or poor communications have introduced long delays in the provision of assistance. The few case examples available suggest that under these conditions, mortality amongst the trapped or seriously injured will be high, and that the need for organized intervention will fall off rapidly with time [see chap. 1, p. 17, chap. 3, p. 86].

These points have five main implications for the immediate supply of relief from international sources:

(1) Assistance with search-and-rescue activities may be required where disaster has struck in remote areas, has cut communications or where people may be trapped under buildings of substantial construction. Effective intervention will generally require specialized skills and/or transport, e.g. helicopters, not unskilled labour.

(2) Substantial international assistance with the treatment of the injured is likely to be required only after earthquakes.

(3) To be of value to survivors, relief assistance must be at the site of need – which is often far from the main airport of a country – within at most, 3–5 days of the impact.

(4) After earthquakes, the types of material required will be for the treatment of injuries which may be in short supply within the affected area (i.e. chiefly analgesics, anesthetics, antibiotics, casting materials, X-ray film, splints, etc.). There is no evidence to suggest that there will be any substantial increase in the needs for other types of drugs and medical supplies for routine use[4].

(5) The total quantity of medical assistance required, even after a major earthquake, will be, relative to the quantity often supplied, small. Even after a major earthquake causing 50,000 injuries, a rough calculation suggests that the total increased requirement of material would amount to no more than perhaps 10 tons in weight[5].

The importance of these points is illustrated by figure 2 which shows the numbers of casualties presenting at hospitals in Guatemala City after

---

[4] The arrival of large numbers of relief teams may increase drug consumption considerably, particularly in areas of the developing world where services are, in normal times, poor. In past relief operations, much cost and effort have been expended on the treatment of chronic and endemic disease unrelated to the effects of the disaster [e.g. 9].

[5] Based on the crude assumptions that of each 1,000 injuries, 50–100 will require intravenous fluids or the application of a cast or splint, but not including the supply of emergency medical facilities.

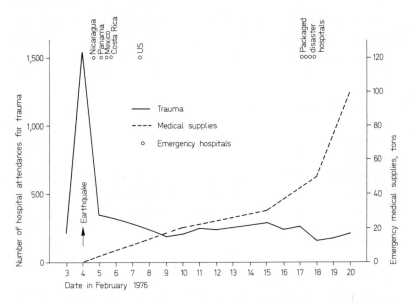

Fig. 2. The number of cases of trauma attending hospitals in Guatemala City and the arrival of medical supplies and emergency hospitals from international donors after the 1976 Guatemala earthquake. Data on hospital attendances calculated from graphs in *Campbell and Spencer* [4]; data on medical supplies from *Mendieta and Moore* [15]; *de Ville de Goyet* et al. [37], and *de Ville de Goyet* [38].

the 1976 earthquake, contrasted with the arrival in the country of medical assistance from abroad. It can be seen that most casualties had been treated, and attendance at hospitals had fallen to normal long before the bulk of supplies had arrived in the country.

The sheer quantities of material supplied and the poor standards of packaging and labeling of drugs in this relief operation also obstructed medical work. *Long* [14], writing of the period immediately after the earthquake observed that 'the level of frustration needed to be seen to be believed. Clinics and hospitals were screaming for more antibiotics and plaster bandages. There were more than enough of the things they needed in the warehouse, but there was no way to get at them'. Also, in spite of the vast quantities of drugs supplied, *de Ville de Goyet* et al. [36] noted that although no acute shortages of drugs were observed even in outlying posts 4 days after the earthquake, some items, including benzathine penicillin, disposable syringes and needles, casting material (which was also lacking in the US emergency field hospital) and sterile gauze and bandages were intermittently in short supply. The material supplied included a 'significant percentage' of time-expired drugs, samples and even previously used perfusion sets.

Figure 2 also shows the time of arrival of various field hospitals after the earthquake. Not suprisingly, those hospitals in place first were military hospitals with self-supporting teams from neighboring countries. The 100-bed US field hospital was operating 4 days after the earthquake but admitted only approximately 200 patients; bed occupancy did not exceed 80%. The 'packaged disaster hospitals', originally intended for use after nuclear war in the US, arrived 14 days after the earthquake, long after a surplus of hospital beds was available in the capital.

The deployment of US emergency medical teams and hospitals after the 1972 earthquake in Nicaragua, which destroyed much of Managua, the capital, also provides a good illustration of the speed with which services must be supplied if they are to be of value. The earthquake occurred at 00.28 a.m. on December 23, and caused an estimated 20,000 injuries. The first US medical team arrived 13 h after the earthquake, and operating outside one of the damaged hospitals in the city saw a total of 300 patients before being replaced by the USAF '1st Tac' hospital at 4 p.m. on December 24, 40 h after the earthquake. By December 25 the patient load had peaked. The hospital was closed on December 29 having seen a total of 900 patients and conducted 44 major surgical operations and applied 200 casts. The US army 21st Evacuation Hospital became operational on December 26, 3 days after the earthquake: 'At the time the 21st Evacuation Hospital became fully operational, the need for acute medical care had largely passed'. 'The . . . type of patients more closely paralleled those found in any general hospital . . . as opposed to an acute disaster situation' [6]. After this disaster, a survey of medical warehouses within the country indicated that considerable amounts of medical and surgical supplies were immediately salvagable, although the warehouses were said to have been completely destroyed [38].

There are few other examples where the time of delivery of relief is known. However, a simple consideration of the logistics of supply from international sources would suggest that the timing of response seen after these disasters in relation to needs is not unusual. Under conditions where disaster has affected a large remote area with few medical services, the problem may be almost insuperable. For example, *Rennie* [23], involved with relief work in Peru in 1970, arrived in the country 6 days after the earthquake and found that 'the problem was simple; to bring immediate succour to the injured, the homeless, the hungry – but how many, where and how?'. The earthquake affected principally the remote highlands of the country, and in the capital, Lima, he found that 'Rumours of 300,000 injured were flying around. Yet so far they had seen scarcely a dozen'. 'Random teams of foreign doctors (112 Argentinians for example) looking for work. In Lima there was clearly no need for my team from Chicago, but the situation in the valley was more obscure. I needed to get up there and find out but there was still no transport'.

In this relief operation, large numbers of helicopters were available from a US aircraft carrier, but these could not reach the high altitudes in the affected areas of the Andes. Only 83 people were admitted to the 300-bed hospital of the aircraft carrier. When relief began to filter into the affected area, and a survey was organized, it was found that although there was immense destruction, there were few serious injuries requiring treatment [23]. The immediate requirements were for water containers, piping, small implements and tools and building materials, which were not available [9].

Environmental Exposure: Emergency Shelter

Disaster-affected populations have proved to be remarkably adept at protecting themselves against environmental exposure, even in cold and wet conditions, chiefly by the use of alternative buildings and by building temporary shelters. On theoretical grounds, a substantial risk of death from exposure appears to be confined to the period during and for some hours after some disasters [see chap. 3].

During the past decade, many studies have been done of the provision of shelter after disaster in both the industrialized and developing countries [7]. These studies raise many issues relevant to the provision of emergency shelter and to reconstruction which are beyond the scope of this book, including land tenure, building styles and technologies appropriate to the social and economic conditions of the individuals and populations concerned. From the narrow perspective of the immediate provision of relief with the object of preventing death from environmental exposure, two points may be made: (1) The conditions under which a population is likely to face a substantial risk of exposure [see chap. 3], the short period for which these conditions persist, the enormous areas and populations which may be affected, and the lack of information about the location of people in need, all argue against any practical possibility of systematic organized intervention to effectively assist survivors. (2) At a later stage after disaster, and depending upon an assessment of the actual needs of the population, international assistance may play an important role in the provision of building materials, e.g. reinforced polythene, to upgrade the quality of temporary shelters, tents of an appropriate design, or financial assistance towards the costs of reconstruction.

Records of the provision of emergency shelter after disasters suggests that except where shelter is available from local sources, protracted delays in supply are common. For example, after the 1970 Peru earthquake (when 500,000 people were estimated to be homeless), 12,400 tents were erected in 10 weeks; after the 1972 Nicaraguan earthquake (200,000 estimated homeless), 40 tents were erected after 2 days, although a 'full compliment' of tents was not available for 5 weeks [see also p. 84]; after the 1975 Lice earthquake in Turkey (5,000 estimated homeless) some tents were supplied within 2 days by the local Red Crescent Society and most of the tents required within 2 weeks. After this earthquake, international emergency housing (polyurethane foam igloos) was not erected for 60 days [35].

Communicable Disease and Disease Control

This topic has already been discussed at length [see chap. 2]: the chief conclusion to emerge is that epidemics are not a potential risk after most disasters, even in the developing countries, except where a population has been displaced into an area without adequate services, or where there has been disruption of water supply or a deterioration in sanitary conditions. The logical approach to communicable disease control after disaster is therefore: (1) To direct attention to the problems of water supply and sanitation for those parts of the population where the potential for disease spread may have increased. Immunization programmes may be required under some defined conditions, e.g., against measles. (2) To institute a system of disease surveillance, so that if outbreaks occur, they can be identified and dealt with appropriately.

Under no circumstances should vaccines be supplied or vaccination programmes begun before their need has been accurately determined.

Food Relief

Short-lived food shortages, resulting from burying household stocks, and the disruption of transportation and marketing systems are a regular consequence of major disasters, regardless of type. Although there are few modern examples, more serious food shortages may result from disasters in which a population has lost food stocks, capital goods, or where long-term unemployment has occurred.

Food distribution may therefore be required for part of a population after many disasters, at least for a short period. Appropriate relief measures for larger affected populations may include government market intervention to prevent price rises, the distribution of cash or the provision of work for the affected population. The necessary stocks of food for short-term distribution may often be found within the affected country, and needs for the urgent importation of food after disasters appears to be rare. There may more frequently be a need to import food to make up stocks at a later date.

In summary therefore, current evidence suggests that the immediate response to a major disaster in a developing country, in the period before accurate information is available as to the specific needs of the population, should be confined to: (1) specialized transport and rescue skills where there is a prima facie case that these are required, and where these can be operational within the probable period of need, i.e. rarely longer than 5 days from the impact; (2) after a major earthquake, medical supplies of a quality and quantity likely to be relevant to the treatment of the injured, if these can be supplied within a similar period. The supply of all other assistance should await a more formal assessment of the needs of survivors.[6]

In some cases, this pattern of response might still exceed the requirements of the affected population. Nevertheless, if adopted, it would substantially reduce the bulk of material supplied and thereby reduce one of the main current obstacles to the speedy and effective supply of relief; it would also potentially free substantial resources for more considered investment in rehabilitation and reconstruction, the costs of which are currently borne chiefly by the developing countries themselves.[7]

---

[6] The question arises as to how this could be implemented, given the current organization of the international relief system. It is probable that several approaches to the problem are required: (1) voluntary restraint by the major relief donors; (2) more effective central coordination; (3) the development within disaster-prone countries of the skills required to assess relief needs and to anticipate the problems which may arise with emergency assistance. For a discussion of this problem see ref. 19.

[7] Estimates by the US Government Office of Foreign Disaster Assistance suggest that, in the period 1965–1975, the ratio of the costs of disaster relief provided from international sources to that provided by the affected countries was 1:42 [19].

Relief After the Emergency Period: The Assessment of Needs

As has been said, the main administrative problem after a major disaster is likely to be a lack of accurate information on the extent and effects of the disaster, the needs of survivors and the resources available for relief.

There is now sufficient practical experience to show that, after most disasters, it should be possible to accurately determine the relief needs. Admittedly, there are few published examples where this has been done: the survey by *Rennie* [23] after the 1970 Peru earthquake; the surveys by *Sommer and Mosely* [24] after the 1970 Bangladesh cyclone/storm surge disaster; the collection of statistics on bed occupancy after various earthquakes [see chap. 1, p. 22]; surveys of water systems and the four examples of disease surveillance outlined in chapter 2. However, the techniques employed – essentially the use of sample and systematic surveys and the establishment of simple reporting systems – are methodologically straightforward, and there is every reason to suppose that, given suitable personnel and transport, reasonably accurate estimates of relief needs could be obtained very quickly after most disasters. Problems may arise with the interpretation of data, particularly in the developing countries, when predisaster 'baseline' levels are unknown, and with the interpretation of incomplete data [see chap. 1, p. 27]. However, most needs assessment is concerned with estimating unambiguous disaster effects, e.g. damage, casualties, or the identification of large changes, such as outbreaks of disease, and in practise these problems do not appear to create much difficulty. It may sometimes be possible to use an adjacent unaffected area as a control. The problems of information collection and interpretation are considerably eased if basic information on population distribution, communications and major health problems are maintained as part of a predisaster plan [20].

Several different schemes have been proposed for the assessment of relief needs after disasters [17, 20, 25]. In practise, the requirements for information will vary with the type of disaster, and the opportunities to collect information with the availability of transport and personnel, and some ingenuity and adaptation of techniques will be needed. Three main types of information collection will be required:

(1) Within the first few days of a disaster, estimates will be required of the geographical extent of the disaster, the size of the affected population, the number of injured, the needs for evacuation and urgent needs for food

and shelter. Information will also be required on the location and condition of medical facilities and on the medical supplies and transport available within the area, in order to project requirements for further assistance with relief. To obtain these estimates, a ground survey, ideally using helicopters, and overflights of the area will usually be required.[8]

(2) As soon as communications permit, these first rapid estimates may be supplemented by regular reports from medical facilities and other relief centers. The information obtained should include the numbers of injured and other diagnostic categories of patients attending medical facilities, the number of admissions, bed occupancy and the requirements for drugs and other supplies. This reporting system will subsequently form the basis of a disease surveillance system.

(3) As the emergency phase passes, more detailed and carefully sampled surveys will be required to obtain more accurate estimates of needs for building materials, food distribution and other interventions to improve food supply. Systematic surveys will also be required of water supplies and other specific utilities. Such surveys may need to be repeated over long periods to guide the process of reconstruction.

During the period immediately after disaster when no information is available about the needs of the population, the epidemiologist also has an important role to play in providing informed advice about the probable health effects which may arise, in establishing priorities for action and in emphasizing the need for accurate information as the basis for relief decisions.

The value of surveys to assess relief needs is illustrated by the experience of *Sommer and Mosely* [25] who conducted surveys after the 1970 Bangladesh cyclone/storm-surge disaster. The first rapid survey took only 4 days to complete and produced results which were confirmed by a later, more detailed survey [see chap. 1, p. 36]. The first survey was completed as international relief was beginning to enter Dacca, the capital city. The results of this allowed the US Government to divert over $2 million which had been allocated to emergency hospitals to the supply of shelter and clothing. The estimated cost of the second detailed survey was only $10,000.

---

[8] The use of satellites has been proposed for information collection after disasters. However, current techniques do not give sufficiently detailed definition, or the analysis of images takes too long for this to be of use during the emergency period [18].

The epidemiologist is now regarded as a 'legitimate, if not indispensable, element of disaster relief' [4]; there is little doubt that as the value of relief decisions based upon reliable information becomes more widely recognized, the epidemiologist will become one of the most important components of relief operations.

References

1 Alexander, D.: The earthquake of 23 November 1980 in Campania and Basilicata, Southern Italy (International Disaster Institute, London 1981).

2 Anonymous: How tornado was fought and managed; Kheonjhar – an example (Indian Art Press, Calcutta 1982).

3 Arnold, C.; Eisner, R.; Durkin, M.; Whitaker, D.: Occupant behaviour in a six-storey office building following severe earthquake damage. Disasters 6: 207–214 (1982).

4 Campbell, C.C.; Spencer, H.C.: Epidemiological assessment of earthquake relief, Guatemala (Center for Disease Control, Atlanta, unpubl. report, 1976).

5 Cohen, S.P.; Raghavulu, C.V.: The Andhra cyclone of 1977 (Vikas Publishing House, New Delhi 1979).

6 Coultrip, R.L.: Medical aspects of US disaster relief operations in Nicaragua. Milit. Med. 139: 879–883 (1974).

7 Davis, I.: Disasters and the small dwelling (Pergamon Press, Oxford 1981).

8 Gaur, S.D.; Marwah, S.M.: Public health aspects of floods with illustrations from 1967 Varanasi floods. Indian J. publ. Hlth. 12: 93–94 (1968).

9 Glass, R.I.: Pishtacos in Peru. Harvard Med. Alum. Bull. 12: 12–16 (1971).

10 Glass, R.I.; Urrutia, J.J.; Siborny, S.; Smith, H.: Earthquake injuries related to housing in a Guatemalan village. Science, N.Y. 197: 638–643 (1977).

11 Glass, R.I.; Craven, R.B.; Bregman, D.J.; Stoll, B.J.; Horowitz, N.; Kerndt, P.; Winckle, J.: Injuries from the Wichita Falls tornado – implications for prevention. Science, N.Y. 207: 734–738 (1980).

12 Green, S.: International disaster relief; towards a responsive system (McGraw-Hill, New York 1977).

13 Haas, J.E.: The Philippine earthquake and tsunami disaster – a reexamination of some behavioural propositions. Disasters 2: 3–9 (1978).

14 Long, E.C.: Sermons in stones – some medical aspects of the earthquake in Guatemala. St. Mary's Hosp. Gaz. Lond. 83: 6–9 (1977).

15 Mendieta, E.; Moore, J.: Activities of pharmacy team in Guatemalan earthquake relief (unpubl. 1976).

16 Michaelis, A.: Disaster past and future (The Daily Telegraph, London, Oct. 1972).

17 National Research Council: Assessing international disaster needs (National Academy of Sciences, Washington 1979).

18 National Research Council: The role of technology in international disaster assistance (National Academy of Sciences, Washington 1978).

19 National Research Council: The US Government foreign disaster assistance program (National Academy of Sciences, Washington 1978).

20   Pan American Health Organization: Emergency health management after natural disaster. Scient. publ. No. 407 (Pan American Health Organization, Washington 1981).

21   Pan American Health Organization: Emergency vector control after natural disaster. Scient. publ. No. 419 (Pan American Health Organization, Washington 1982).

22   Quarantelli, E.L.: The community general hospital: its immediate problems in disasters. Am behav. Scient. *13:* 380; cited in Western, K.A.: The epidemiology of natural and man-made disasters – the present state of the art; thesis University of London (1972).

23   Rennie, D.: After the earthquake. Lancet *i:* 704–707 (1970).

24   Sommer, A.; Mosely, W.H.: East Bengal cyclone of November 1970 – epidemiological approach to disaster assessment. Lancet *ii:* 1029–1036 (1972).

25   Sommer, A.; Mosely, W.H.: The cyclone: medical assessment and determination of relief; in Chen, Disaster in Bangladesh: health crises in a developing nation (Oxford University Press, New York 1973).

26   United Nations Disaster Relief Coordinator: Report on the earthquakes in Irian Jaya and Bali, Indonesia, June–July 1976 (UNDRO, Geneva 1976).

27   United Nations Disaster Relief Coordinator: Report on the floods in Mozambique, February 1977 (UNDRO, Geneva 1977).

28   United Nations Disaster Relief Coordinator: Report on the cyclone and torrential rains in the Sultanate of Oman, June 1977 (UNDRO, Geneva 1977).

29   United Nations Disaster Relief Coordinator: Report on the earthquake in Van Province, Turkey, 24 November 1976 (UNDRO, Geneva 1977).

30   United Nations Disaster Relief Coordinator: Report on the cyclone in Sri Lanka, November 23/24, 1978 (UNDRO, Geneva 1979).

31   United Nations Disaster Relief Coordinator: Report on the floods in Jamaica, June 1979 (UNDRO, Geneva 1980).

32   United Nations Disaster Relief Coordinator: Report on hurricane David in Dominica August 29, 1979 (UNDRO, Geneva 1980).

33   United Nations Disaster Relief Coordinator: Report on hurricanes David and Frederick in the Dominican Republic, August/September 1979 (UNDRO, Geneva 1980).

34   United Nations Disaster Relief Coordinator: Report on the earthquake in Kerman province (Iran) 28 July 1981 (UNDRO, Geneva 1981).

35   United Nations Disaster Relief Coordinator: Shelter after disaster; guidelines for assistance (United Nations, New York 1982).

36   de Ville de Goyet, C.; del Cid, E.; Romero, A.; Jeanee, E.; Lechat, M.: Earthquake in Guatemala – epidemiological evaluation of the relief effort. Bull. Pan. Am. Hlth Org. *10:* 95–109 (1976).

37   de Ville de Goyet, C.; Lechat, M.F.; Boucquey, C.: Drugs and supplies for disaster relief. Trop. Doct. *6:* 168–170 (1976).

38   Ville de Goyet, C., de; Assessment of health needs and priorities. Joint IHF/IUA/UNDRO/WHO Seminar, Manila 1978; cited in [17].

39   Ville de Goyet, C., de; Seaman, J.; Geijer, U.: The management of nutritional emergencies in large populations (World Health Organization, Geneva 1978).

40   Western, K.A.: Epidemiologic surveillance after natural disaster. Scient. publ. No. 420 (Pan American Health Organization, Washington 1982).

Appendix: Volcanoes

J. Seaman, C. Hogg

This topic has been presented in an appendix because of the comparative rarity of volcanic eruption as a cause of disasters and because, as yet, few useful statements can be made about their effects on health. There is wide variation in the effects of volcanoes, and any given volcano may change its character over time or even during the course of one eruption. Most scientific efforts in this area have been directed towards the development of methods for monitoring and predicting eruptions, to allow the timely evacuation of the populations at risk, and towards methods of reducing damage, (e.g., by the diversion of lava flows).

In comparison with other types of disaster, mortality from volcanic action is low. It is estimated that, during the last 500 years, only about 200,000 people (400/year) have died from this cause [17]. However, because of the fertility of volcanic soils, the areas around many volcanoes are densely populated, and within these areas the risks may be substantial. For example, more than a million people live in the area around Merapi volcano in central Java, and 'every few decades eruptions take from a few hundred to a few thousand lives' [17].

Much of the world's volcanic activity occurs along the margins of the major tectonic plates [see chap. 1, p. 10], therefore coinciding with areas of high earthquake risk: the vast majority of the 760 [22] currently active volcanoes are to be found in the countries bordering the Pacific ocean (the 'ring of fire'), through Indonesia (the 'Sundra arc'), in the West Indies, Iceland, the eastern Mediterranean and in East and Central Africa. The exceptions to this rule are the Himalayas and much of the northern Indian subcontinent, where earthquakes are common but which are almost devoid of volcanic activity, and Hawaii, where the reverse is the case. However, the term 'active' volcano may be misleading as volcanoes may erupt after long periods of quiescence or when they are thought to be extinct, e.g. Tristan da Cunha, which erupted in 1961.

This review has been divided into two parts: (1) a general review of types of volcanic activity and their effects on health; (2) summaries of the few case examples where aspects of effects of volcanic activity on health have been studied in detail.

Types of Volcanic Activity and Their Effects on Health

Volcanoes may affect the health of populations in two main ways: directly, from blast, lava flows, ash and other effects; and indirectly, by causing tsunamis [see p. 38], population movements and adverse effects on agriculture. This section is chiefly based on a review by UNDRO [7].

Direct Effects of Volcanic Activity

Two main variables determine the characteristics of a volcanic eruption: the fluidity or viscosity of the lava and the extent of the gas pressure. Briefly, the more viscous the lava and the higher the gas pressure built up before an eruption, the greater the potential hazard. Volcanic activity ranges from a gentle outpouring of lava to violent explosions which throw great volumes of rock high into the atmosphere. This activity can be categorized under six main headings: (1) lava flows, (2) domes, (3) tephra, (4) glowing avalanches, (5) lahars, and (6) volcanic gases. Any given volcano may exhibit several of these effects.

Lava Flows

The extent, thickness and speed of advance of a lava flow varies with the volume of lava, its fluidity and the topography of the area. The speed of advance of a lava flow varies from only a few metres/day up to 40 kph or more on steeper slopes. However, because the speed of advance is usually slow, lava flows are generally of little risk to life. But as they may cause extensive damage to property, many methods have been tried to control their direction of flow and speed, including aerial high-explosive bombing, the erection of diversion barriers and cooling the advancing edge of the lava flow with water jets.

Domes

Viscous lavas may pile up over their vents to form domes; these grow by expansion from within, and vary in size from a few metres wide and deep to as much as 2000 m wide and 600 m deep. The expansion of a dome results in cracking of the solid exterior carapace, and the more or less continuous displacement of blocks, which roll down and may represent a hazard to people. In some cases, the cooling of viscous magma protruding through fractures in the carapace of the dome forms 'spines', which sometimes reach 100 m in height. These are unstable and may cause avalanches.

Tephra (Pyroclastic Material)

This term includes all material thrown out from volcanic eruptions, ranging in size from dust to blocks several metres across. Larger tephra tends to be deposited close to the vent, whereas dust and ash injected high into the atmosphere may be carried for thousands of kilometres. Rain falling through clouds of ash may form mud balls; the ejection of water from a volcano, with ash and other debris, may result in blankets of mud over large areas.

For descriptive purposes, the effects of tephra have been divided into two parts: the direct physical effects of tephra, and the effects of dust and ash on the respiratory tract and eye.

Direct Effects of Tephra. Falling blocks may start fires or injure animals or people. For example, during the 1968 eruption of Arénal, Costa Rica, falling blocks crashed through houses 3 km from the erupting vent. When deposited, ash is seldom hot enough to cause fires. However, the weight of ash may cause the roofs of houses to collapse. In the 1971 eruption of Fuego, Guatemala, a thickness of 30 cm of ash was deposited 8 km west of the volcano and caused the collapse of about one-fifth of the roofs in the town of Yepocapa. During the eruption of Vesuvius in AD 79, many people were killed when buildings collapsed under the weight of ash.

Long continued ash producing eruptions may necessitate evacuation of the population from the area, although examples of this are rare. Two further types of ash eruption are the base surge and the ash flow. The base surge forms in the base of some volcano columns. It consists of a ring-shaped cloud of suspended ash expanding at great speed, eroding the surface near the vent. In the inner zone, trees may be broken off or uprooted, and buildings raised. At a greater range, objects may be severely sand-blasted. In some eruptions, much of the ash remains suspended in a cloud and moves close to the ground, an effect known as an ash flow. Friction is eliminated by expanding gas within the cloud, which holds the particles of ash apart. The flow is propelled by gravity, and follows the topography of the ground; ash flows may sometimes exceed 200 kph in velocity.

Effects of Ash on the Respiratory Tract and Eyes. Five factors are important in assessing the health risks from ashfall: the airborne concentration of total suspended particles; the size of the particles; the frequency and duration of exposure; host factors such as preexisting respiratory disease; and the presence of crystalline silica (SiO_2) in the ash.

People may be asphyxiated by volcanic ash. In Pompeii, (buried in the eruption of Vesuvius in AD 79) some excavated victims were found covering their faces with their hands, or with cloth, presumably asphyxiated by ash. More recently, several deaths were caused in this way during the eruption of Mount St. Helens, Washington State, USA. This example is discussed at length below.

Exposure to airborne crystalline silica of a respirable size, i.e., less than 10 µm particle diameter, which can enter the alveoli of the lung, may lead to airway irritation and to symptoms of airway obstruction. If the exposure is at a sufficiently high concentration and for a long enough time, silicosis may result, a disabling and sometimes fatal pulmonary fibrosis, usually seen as an industrial disease. As volcanic ash may contain crystalline silica of a respirable size, this is of some interest as both an acute and long-term problem for ash-exposed populations: the few relevant published studies are summarized later in this review.

Particles of ash may enter the eyes as 'foreign bodies' and cause corneal abrasions or conjunctivitis.

Glowing Avalanches (Nuées Ardentes, Pyroclastic Flows)

Three main types are recognized, named for the volcanoes in which each effect was first observed (Soufrière, Merapi and Pelée). Although there are different mechanisms by which each of these is formed, their effects are similar: a turbulent mass of superheated gas, with dust, hot ash and lava fragments, travelling at speeds of up to 160 kph and killing everything in its path. The glowing avalanche which struck the town of St. Pierre, Martinique in 1902 killed all but 2 of the 28,000 inhabitants of the town.

Lahars

This term covers many types of volcanic mudflow. These vary in temperature from cold to boiling. Propelled by gravity they can achieve speeds of 100 kph, travel considerable distances and cover areas of up to several hundred square kilometres. Lahars are common, and are the major cause of volcanic destruction and loss of life. Lahars may arise from the ejection of water from a crater lake, from snow melt, by the displacement of water-saturated ash or soil down the slope of a volcano, and in many other ways in which volcanic activity interacts with water. As lahars can travel at considerable speed, substantial mortality may result. For example, at Kelud, Java in 1919, 5,000 people were killed by a lahar and several hundred square kilometres of land was lost.

Rarely, a lahar may contain a sufficient concentration of sulphuric or hydrochloric acid to cause chemical burning of exposed skin. One such instance resulted from the explosion of the crater lake of Kawah Idjen, Java in 1917.

Volcanic Gases

Gases given off by volcanic action contain, in various proportions, water vapour, carbon dioxide, carbon monoxide, sulphur dioxide, sulphur trioxide, hydrogen sulphide, hydrogen chloride, hydrogen fluoride, methane and more complex hydrocarbons as well as nitrogen, argon and other inert gases. These can affect people in various ways. Carbon dioxide and sulphur dioxide may cause asphyxiation: the former by its accumulation in 'pools' in low lying areas, the latter by its direct effects on the respiratory tract. Sheep, wild animals and birds have been asphyxiated by carbon dioxide after volcanic eruptions, e.g., after the Hekla, Iceland eruption of 1947, although deaths of human beings are rare. During the 1973 eruption of Eldafell, Iceland, the only human death occurred when a man sought shelter in a cellar filled with carbon dioxide and was asphyxiated. Before the destruction of St. Pierre Martinique in 1902, concentrations of sulphur dioxide in the town were reported to be sufficient to cause the death of horses [22].

Secondary Effects of Volcanic Eruptions

The most serious consequences of volcanic eruption may arise from secondary effects, principally from tsunami [see chap. 1, p. 38], from population movements and from indirect effects on agriculture.

Tsunami

In 1883, the uninhabited island of Krakatoa in the Indian Ocean exploded and caused a tsunami which killed over 30,000 people along the coasts of Java and Sumatra. In remoter history, other examples can be found, including the destructive tsunami caused by the eruption which led to the formation of the island of Santorini in the eastern Mediterranean in about 1500 BC.

Population Movements

Volcanic eruption, or the threat of an eruption, may cause the displacement of populations or their evacuation by government authorities. As with any refugee population, this may cause problems with water and food supply, sanitation, and increase the risks of the transmission of communicable diseases. After the May 1982 eruption of El Chinchonal volcano, Mexico, 140,000 people were reported to have been evacuated by the government [21]. *Gueri* et al. [13] describe the management of food supply in evacuation centres after the 1979 eruption of La Soufrière volcano, St. Vincent in the Caribbean.

Effects on Agriculture, Livestock and Food Production

Volcanic activity may lead to adverse effects on livestock and on agriculture, either at close range to a volcano or at greater distances. In rare instances, famine has resulted.

Ash may affect livestock in several ways. It may kill pasture through direct physical action; grazing animals may die from ingestion of large quantities of ash, e.g., at Kodiak, Alaska in 1912; or, they may be poisoned by the toxic constituents of the ash. During the 1947 and 1970 eruptions of Hekla, Iceland, fluorine poisoning caused the deaths of thousands of sheep. Experiments showed that grass with a fluorine concentration of as little as 250 ppm was sufficient to kill sheep. One case of cobalt poisoning of sheep in New Zealand was traced of an ash layer of prehistoric age.

Direct damage to crops may occur by ash loads which may break branches off of trees, or acid deposits which may destroy leaves. Following the 1783 Laki eruption in Iceland, the countryside for hundreds of square miles around was covered in sulphurous fumes, affecting livestock and crops. This led to what became known as the 'haze famine' in which 20% of the population are said to have died [22]. In 1815, the eruption of Tambora, Java, caused widespread destruction of crops and reportedly killed over 80,000 people. The same volcano led to climatic changes which caused famine as far away as New England a year later [20].

As might be expected, the chemical emissions from volcanoes have complex biological effects. A bibliography of relevant references is given by the US National Library of Medicine [16]. One recently discovered effect is an association between volcanic soils and endemic, non-filarial elephantiasis, in East Africa. This is due to lymphatic obstruction secondary to the absorption of crystalline amorphous silica directly through the exposed skin [18].

Case Examples

Mount St. Helens, Washington State, USA

A considerable amount of information is available on morbidity and mortality resulting from this eruption, from studies by epidemiologists from the US Center for Disease Control.

The eruption of Mount St. Helens, on May 18, 1980, was preceded by an avalanche on the north side of the mountain, triggered by an earthquake. The resulting lateral explosion blew out a large section of the mountainside and affected a wide area, approximately a 180° arc to the north of the mountain. This area can be roughly divided into three parts: an inner area, affected by a mudflow, to a radius of approximately 6 km from the crater, and draining northwest down a river valley; an area designated the 'tree blown-down area', also forming roughly the shape of an arc extending to a depth of approximately 15 km beyond the mudflow; and an outer fringe zone 2–3 km in depth in which trees were left standing but were killed by the blast (the 'tree destruction area').

In addition to the effects of blast and mudflow, huge quantities of ash were thrown out both during and subsequent to the main explosion. By October 16, 1980, six eruptions had occurred, distributing ash over wide areas of Washington and neighbouring states.

Mortality [11]

By August 1980, 29 bodies had been recovered. 2 persons were rescued and subsequently died of complications from burns, and 32 people were listed as missing. Some of these were known to have been in the area affected by mudflow, pyroclastic flow and heavy ashfall. Survivors of the eruption were interviewed to determine their exact location at the time of the blast. This group was defined as persons who had been within approximately 8 km of Mount St. Helens, or the areas affected by tree destruction during the May 18 eruption. 100 people met this criterion, but only 53 of these were within 1 mile (1.6 km) of the tree destruction zone. Most of the remaining 47 had been located to the southwest and southeast of the mountain, away from the direction of the blast.

No bodies were recovered from an arbitrarily-defined 'blast area' in the lee of the north side of the mountain. As parts of this area were covered by the mudflow, bodies might not have been found.

In the 'tree blown-down area', roughly 30 km from east to west and 15 km from north to south, 25 bodies were found. 2 survivors were also found in this area, although they subsequently died. The causes of death in this group included trauma (n = 6), asphyxia from smoke and ash (n = 16), and severe burns (n = 3). The deaths from trauma resulted from severe blast (n = 1), a fall (n = 1), flying rock (n = 1), and falling trees (n = 3). The person killed by a rock was located inside an automobile. Of the 15 who died from asphyxia and ash inhalation, 7 were inside vehicles, 4 were adjacent to vehicles and 4 were not near vehicles.

11 survivors, all of whom were at the edge of the 'tree blown-down area' sustained fractures (n = 1), third-degree burns (n = 2), second-degree burns (n = 2), or were unharmed (n = 6) except for possible ash inhalation. Only 3 of this group (2 of whom had second-degree burns) were inside a vehicle.

In the 'tree destruction area', 2 bodies were recovered after the May 18 blast: 1 person found inside a vehicle had died of asphyxia; the other had burns from what might have been a gasoline fire. 2 of the 6 survivors in this area were not under shelter and suffered second- to third-degree burns, even though they were over 15 miles (24 km) northeast of the volcano. The other 4 survivors in this area escaped unharmed in cars.

Within 1 mile of the area of tree destruction, 2 persons died from asphyxia and ash inhalation in and beside automobiles. In this area, none of the 36 survivors suffered serious injuries.

On a typical working day, there are usually approximately 1,000 loggers in the area around Mount St. Helens; the explosion occurred on a Sunday when most of them were away.

Problems Related to Ashfall

Four effects were observed: (1) an increase in acute respiratory illness; (2) eye problems associated with ash; (3) an increase in accidents; (4) a possible pneumoconiosis risk from ash inhalation.

Acute Respiratory Illness

Soon after the eruption of May 18, a hospital-based surveillance system was established in affected parts of Washington state. In general, areas which had experienced high ashfall also experienced an increased number of emergency-room visits and hospital admissions for respiratory illnesses in the 2-week period following the ashfall, and by the 3rd or 4th week, rates of attendance had returned roughly to pre-eruption rates. Areas with moderate ashfall showed little or no increase in visits for pulmonary diseases. The greatest increase in attendance was seen in areas with the highest ashfall.

Measurements of total suspended particulates (TSP) in the air were conducted at ten monitoring stations within the ashfall area. After the first eruption on May 18, peak levels of TSP at three stations were in the range 13,860–35,809 $\mu g/m^3$ [2]. At Addy in Washington state, 24-hour average levels of TSP were 4,059 $\mu g/m^3$ after the eruption of May 18, which caused an ashfall of ⅛ inch, and 13,212 $\mu g/m^3$ after the eruption of July 22 when ¼ inch of ash fell [9]. US Environmental Protection Agency ambient air quality standards for 24-hour average exposure range from a 'primary' level of 260 $\mu g/m^3$ through 'alert', at 375 $\mu g/m^3$; 'warning' 625 $\mu g/m^3$; 'emergency' 875 $\mu g/m^3$ to 'significant harm' at 1,000 $\mu g/m^3$ [8]. These standards, however, are set for industrial particulate emissions usually associated with sulphur dioxide and other pollutants. To assess the potential effects on the respiratory system due to volcanic ash, it is necessary to consider both the chemical composition and particle size of the ash [see p. 160]. Variations in attendance at locations with similar amounts of ashfall could be accounted for by variations in the composition of the ash and by the amount of rainfall in the different areas following the eruption.

By June 3, 1980, sulphur dioxide emissions from the volcano were estimated at 100–200 tons/day. By June 6, this had increased to 1,000 tons/day. However, monitoring showed that there was no increase in sulphur dioxide above background levels in the ambient air [4].

A review of the medical records of 200 patients attending two hospitals at Yakima, 85 miles (136 km) from the mountain, which received over 1 inch of ash after the May 18 eruption, showed that although some of the increase in attendance was due to anxiety and apprehension, most patients had objective clinical signs. Patients with asthma, the largest category of increased visits, had symptoms of cough, dyspnoea, and wheezing, although only a small number required hospitalisation. An increased incidence of bronchitis was found, predominantly in younger age groups, with wheezing as the major clinical sign. Although only a small increase was noted in attendance for patients with pre-existing respiratory disease, patients with chronic obstructive pulmonary disease and emphysema were, in terms of hospitalisation rates, the most severely affected [9].

Overall, only a modest increase in attendance occurred. At Yakima, total hospital attendance for all types of respiratory diagnosis nearly doubled in the 2-week period following the eruption, compared to the 2-week period immediately prior to the eruption (232 vs. 122) [9]. At Moses Lake, which received a very heavy ashfall (2–3 inches), emergency-room visits increased by approximately 35% the week after eruption, and admission by approximately 5% [1].

Preliminary results of a sample survey of approximately 4% of all residents in the Moses Lake area showed an increase in coughs and mild irritation of the eyes, nose and throat in the 2 weeks following the eruption. Haemoptysis was reported by 2 people, both of whom had been heavily exposed to ash [3].

Eye Problems

Increased hospital attendance for eye complaints was also noted. In Yakima, two types of ash fell: large coarse granules resembling grey sand, and a fine grey powder. Increased numbers of emergency-room visits were found for corneal abrasion, foreign bodies in the eye, eye irritation and conjunctivitis or 'red eye'. As with respiratory complaints, eye complaints were found to be most marked in the 2 weeks after an eruption. However, of 129 patients complaining of eye problems, only 42 (33%) were judged to be related to ash exposure [10].

A random telephone survey in three towns in Washington state showed that 4–8% of those sampled reported eye irritation after ashfall. However, only 10–11% of those affected visited a physician as a result.

Accidents

A number of ash-related injuries were noted at Moses Lake, including motor vehicle accidents and falls from ladders, as residents attempted to clear ash from the roofs of their homes.

Pneumoconiosis Risk

Between June 3 and 13, 1980, environmental and personal air samples were collected in five Washington state communities and one in northern Idaho that were exposed to ash from the May 18 or 25 eruptions, with the object of assessing occupational exposures and community concentrations of respirable dust ($< 10\,\mu m$ particle size). The average respirable dust concentration from eleven categories of exposed workers, including clean-up crews, forestry and agricultural workers and the police was 0.4 mg/m³ (range 0.05–0.67 mg/m³). Four area samples from homes, schools, commercial establishments and automobiles averaged 0.07 mg/m³ (range 0.03–0.1 mg/m³) [6]. Those occupations which had an average respirable dust concentration of 0.45 mg/m³ or more exceeded 0.8 mg/m³ from 15 to 31% of the time [6]. Analysis of ash of respirable particle size obtained from three settled dust samples showed that these contained 6% of free crystalline silica [3].

The US recommended limit for occupational exposure to free silica in 50 μg/m³ [6]. With the qualification that this limit was designed for occupational exposure and was not designed for exposure to volcanic ash, an approximate 'permitted exposure limit' was calculated[1] [5]. Respirable dust concentrations of 0.8–1.0 mg/m³ containing 5–6% free silica would yield approximately 50μg free silica/m³ air. It was concluded that, based on available epidemiological data, nearly all occupationally-exposed workers could be exposed to this concentration for 8 hours a day, 5 days a week for many years without being expected to develop silicosis. During the sampling period, some clean-up crews, rubbish workers and forest workers were exposed to concentrations of respirable dust that exceeded 0.8 mg/m³ 15–31% of the time. Recommendations were made for respirator use by heavily-exposed workers [6].

It was concluded that if there were further ashfall or sustained work in heavy ashfall which would result in prolonged exposure over a period of several years, exposed workers would be at increased risk from silicosis. The very low levels of respirable dust measured in community settings, if these can be considered representative of future exposure, suggested that the general population was not at risk of this disease.

A study by *Green* et al. [12] in which rats were injected intratracheally with ash from the Mount St. Helens' volcano, resulted in an acute pulmonary inflammatory response in the rats followed by a granulomatous and fibrotic reaction persisting to the end of the 6-month study period. The bulk of the ash (99% by count and 81% by weight) was found to be of respirable particle size. The ash contained a range of minerals. Crystal-

---

[1] Where the permitted exposure limit $\approx \dfrac{10}{\%\ \text{free SiO}_2 + 2}$ (mg/m³).

line silica constituted 7.2% of the ash by weight. Post-mortem examination of the lungs of 2 loggers who had been working in the area of Mount St. Helens on the day of the eruption showed intra-alveolar foci in 1, resembling the lesions seen in the animal studies, and in the other, an acute interstitial reaction with clusters of giant cells containing ash in the alveoli. The men died 10 and 16 days after the eruption, respectively. The authors urged caution in the interpretation of these findings, as the rat experiments were based on exposures far higher than those likely to be found in the general population; the human cases were also complicated by other factors, including extensive burns. However, the authors concluded that volcanic ash is moderately fibrogenic and should be considered a pneumoconiosis risk among heavily-exposed individuals. They suggest that precautions be taken to monitor air concentrations of particulate matter in order to minimise ash exposure in those likely to be heavily exposed.

Psychiatric Morbidity [7]

On the day of the eruption residents of Yakima, located 85 miles from the mountain, experienced ashfall accompanied by lightning, thunder and a smell of rotten eggs; for much of the day the town was shrouded in darkness. As few people had been warned of the cloud's impending approach, and none had previously experienced an ashfall, there was considerable anxiety about possible health effects. However, records kept by the Central Washington Comprehensive Mental Health Programme, based on an 'open-line' telephone, showed no increase or unusual problems for May, compared with the 4 pre-eruption months. There was no increase in behavioural and emotional problems, in the number of people requiring emotional support, nor in voluntary or involuntary admissions to the psychiatric ward at Yakima Valley Memorial Hospital.

Irazú Volcano, Costa Rica [14]

Irazu volcano, Costa Rica, erupted intermittently from March 1963, causing heavy ashfall on the capital city San José, approximately 15 miles west of the mountain. Daily records of ashfall in San José showed that the greatest ashfall, of 1,248g m^2 settled on the city on December 3 1963; intense volcanic activity continued until December 6 and then gradually tapered off to modest activity by December 9.

Chemical analysis of the ash showed that about 1% of the ash was present in the form of free silica. Particle sizing and counting by microscope indicated that in two samples, 63% and 64% were ≤ 10 μm in diameter; counts obtained by filtering three samples and re-entraining them into the air gave estimates of 25, 26 and 74% of particles in the same size range.

An air sample taken during an eruption in the period January 24–28, 1964, in San José showed that levels of total suspended particulates were 800 μg/m³ of air. Microscopic examination of this sample showed that about 30% of the particles were less than 5 μm in diameter.

No gas analysis was conducted, although some individuals in San José noted that the taste of sulphur gases was noticeable to a minor extent in the city. The minimum quantity of sulphur dioxide detectable by taste is said to be approximately 0.3 ppm [14].

The effects of ashfall on the population were determined by questioning individuals and physicians in the community. The effects during eruptions and during periods of wind-blown resuspended ash were apparently similar, although the latter were generally less severe.

Acute conjunctivitis with redness and burning of the eyes occurred on exposure to ash, although the effects apparently subsided rapidly when exposure to dust ceased. Throat irritation, sometimes accompanied by a dry cough was common, as was inflammation and burning of the throat; this effect also cleared up within a short time after cessation of exposure. Some persons were also affected by nasal irritation and discharge.

When exposure to ash was combined with upper respiratory infection, the effects were severe and prolonged. A few people developed severe bronchitic symptoms which lasted for some days beyond the period of exposure to the ash. This type of reaction was found particularly in people with pre-existing chest disease, e.g., chronic bronchitis. Local physicians agreed that the effects of ash were not severe enough to cause any deaths, even in those with preexisting disease.

Soufrière Volcano, St. Vincent, West Indies [15]

St. Vincent is located in the Windward Islands in the Caribbean. Early on April 13, 1979, the Soufrière volcano, located in the north of the island, erupted after 10 months of premonitory activity. From April 13 to 26, the volcano went through several explosive phases accompanied by ashfalls, pyroclastic flows and mud flows. The southern part of the island, including Kingstown, the capital, experienced several falls of fine ash. As warning of the eruption was given, evacuation was possible. Some 15,000–20,000 people were evacuated from the area within a 5-km radius of the volcano and assembled in 63 evacuation centres, where they remained for over 2 months. Epidemiological surveillance was organized, including surveillance of hospital admissions to the Kingstown General Hospital, the only functioning general hospital in the island at that time.

During the first week of volcanic activity, it was found that the number of admissions to the paediatric ward increased from approximately 25/week before the eruption to 53 in the week following. The most frequent reason for admission in the week after the volcano was gastroenteritis (n = 15, 28.3%), followed by asthmatic bronchitis (n = 12, 22.6%), respiratory infections (n = 10, 18.9%), accidents (n = 8, 15.1%) and other (n = 8, 15.1%). Before the eruption, the normal rate of admission for asthmatic bronchitis was 0–1/week; during the same month as the eruption in the previous 2 years, there were 1–2 admissions for asthmatic bronchitis each month. In the second week after the eruption, the number of admissions for asthmatic bronchitis fell to 6, and in the third and fourth post-eruption weeks to 1 and 2 cases, respectively. Of the 18 cases of asthmatic bronchitis which occurred in the first 2 post-eruption weeks, no cases occurred in children under the age of 1 year, 10 cases in children aged 1–3 years, 5 cases in children aged 3–5 years and 3 cases in children aged 4–10 years. Both sexes were equally affected.

Several hypotheses were advanced for the increase in admissions for asthmatic bronchitis, including the possibility of faulty diagnosis, epidemic respiratory infections, psychological disturbances related to the evacuation, and exposure to volcanic emissions. The first two of these could be dismissed; the third and fourth could not be assessed. Therefore, no firm conclusion could be drawn.

Sulphur dioxide, sulphur trioxide and hydrogen sulphide were recovered from the volcanic gases, and people were noted to have complained of eye and throat irritation. Heavy ashfall from this volcano also fell on the island of Barbados, 180 km to the east of St. Vincent, on April 13–14, but this was not accompanied by a change in the incidence of asthmatic bronchitis.

Mount Usu Volcano, Hokkaido, Japan 1977

On April 7, 1977, Mount Usu erupted. During the week of August 7–16, 18 eruptions occurred which covered many towns and cities of Hokkaido with 2–17 cm of ash. A survey was carried out several months after the eruption, aimed at identifying associated illnesses. While many health problems were reported, the investigators concluded that only

10–20% of the complaints of cough and eye irritations were attributable to volcanic ash. Primary school children in two areas were followed up to the month of September 1977. The daily prevalence of cough (4–15%), red eye (0–2%), nose irritation (1–5%), and sore throat (3–8%) were generally higher in areas of heavier ashfall [19].

References

1   Center for Disease Control: Mount St. Helens volcano health report No. 2 (Department of Health and Human Services, Center for Disease Control, Atlanta 1980).
2   Center for Disease Control: Mount St. Helens volcano health report No. 3 (Department of Health and Human Services, Center for Disease Control, Atlanta 1980).
3   Falk, H.; Baxter, P.J.; Ing, R.; French, J.; Heath, C.W.; Merchant, J.A.: Mount St. Helens volcano health report No. 7 (Department of Health and Human Services, Center for Disease Control, Atlanta 1980).
4   Falk, H.; Baxter, P.J.; Ing, R.; French, J.; Heath, C.W.; Merchant, J.A.: Mount St. Helens volcano health report No. 9 (Department of Health and Human Services, Center for Disease Control, Atlanta 1980).
5   Falk, H.; Baxter, P.J.; Ing, R.; French, J.; Heath, C.W.; Merchant, J.A.: Mount St. Helens volcano health report No. 11 (Department of Health and Human Services, Center for Disease Control, Atlanta 1980).
6   Falk, H.; Baxter, P.J.; Ing, R.; French, J.; Stein, G.F.; Heath, C.W.; Merchant, J.A.: Mount St. Helens volcano health report No. 12 (Department of Health and Human Services, Center for Disease Control, Atlanta 1980).
7   Falk, H.; Baxter, P.J.; Ing, R.; French, J.; Gary, F.; Stein, G.F.; Heath, C.W.; Merchant, J.A.: Mount St. Helens volcano health report No. 14 (Department of Health and Human Services, Center for Disease Control, Atlanta 1980).
8   Falk, H.; Baxter, P.J.; Ing, R.; Fench, J.; Stein, G.F.; Heath, C.W.; Merchant, J.A.: Mount St. Helens volcano health report No. 15 (Department of Health and Human Services, Center for Disease Control, Atlanta 1980).
9   Falk, H.; Baxter, P.J.; Ing, R.; French, J.; Heath, C.W.; Bernstein, R.; Merchant, J.A.: Mount St. Helens volcano health report No. 17 (Department of Health and Human Services, Center for Disease Control, Atlanta 1980).
10   Falk, H.; Baxter, P.J.; Ing, R.; French, J.; Heath, C.W.; Bernstein, R.; Merchant, J.A.: Mount St. Helens volcano health report No. 18 (Department of Health and Human Services, Center for Disease Control, Atlanta 1980).
11   Falk, H.; Baxter, P.J.; Ing, R.; French, J.; Heath, C.W.; Bernstein, R.; Merchant, J.A.: Mount St. Helens volcano health report No. 19 (Department of Health and Human Services, Center for Disease Control, Atlanta 1980).
12   Green, F.H.W.; Vallythan, V.; Mentnech, M.S.; Tucker, J.H.; Merchant, J.A.: Is volcanic ash a pneumoconiosis risk? Nature, Lond. 293: 216–217 (1981).
13   Gueri, M.; Allen, B.; Iton, M.: Nutritional status of vulnerable groups in evacuation centres during the eruption of La Soufrière volcano in St. Vincent 1979. Disasters 6: 10–15 (1982).

14   Horton, R.J.M.; McCaldin, R.O.: Observations on air pollution aspects of Irazú
      volcano, Costa Rica. Publ. Hlth Rep., Wash. *79:* 925–929 (1964).

15   Leus, X.; Kintanar, C.; Bowman, V.: Asthmatic bronchitis associated with a volcanic
      eruption in St. Vincent, West Indies. Disasters *5:* 67–69 (1981).

16   National Library of Medicine: Biomedical effects of volcanoes. Specialized Bibliography
      Series, SBS No. 1980–1 (National Library of Medicine, US Department of Health and
      Human Services, 1980).

17   Office of the United Nations Disaster Relief Co-ordinator. Disaster prevention and miti-
      gation: a compendium of current knowledge, vol. *1:* Volcanological aspects (United
      Nations, New York 1977).

18   Price, E.W.; Henderson, W.J.: The elemental content of lymphatic tissues of bare-footed
      people of Ethiopia, with reference to endemic elephantiasis of the lower legs. Trans. R.
      Soc. trop. Med. Hyg. *72:* 132–136 (1978).

19   Seki, K.: Usu eruption and its impact on the environment (Hokkaido University,
      December 1978); cited in [10].

20   Stommel, H.; Stommel, E.: The year without a summer. Scient. Am. *240:* 134–140
      (1979).

21   The Guardian: London (April 1, 1982).

22   Whittow, J.: Disasters (Lane, London 1980).

Subject Index